Praise for *Us Against Alzheimer's*

"The stories in this anthology are moving and illuminating. I believe in the power of story to educate and demystify, to demolish fear and shame, to generate conversation and connectedness. To humanize. It is through stories like these that we begin to understand people living with Alzheimer's, and maybe—through empathy and compassion—we can heal what can't yet be cured."

—Lisa Genova, *New York Times*-
bestselling author of *Still Alice*

"Alzheimer's can be isolating and terrifying, but when we share powerful stories like these, we begin to tear down the walls that keep it in the shadows. The powerful voices in this book shine a light full of humanity, heart, and healing to a disease that has affected so many."

—Lauren and Seth Rogen,
Founders of Hilarity For Charity

"This anthology is terrific. It is the perfect read for those who have or have had the Alzheimer's experience. The stories are heartfelt and real, and will make a difference in the lives of many. Another excellent piece of work from Marita Golden!"

—Goldie S. Byrd. Alzheimer's Researcher and Director,
Maya Angelou Center for Health Equity,
Wake Forest School of Medicine

"Here is what's so beautiful about this book: It is chock full of people sticking their necks out and telling their story. With clarity, with patience, with feeling, with faith."

—David Shenk, cohost of the podcast
The Forgetting: Inside the Mind of Alzheimer's,
author of *The Forgetting*, and creator of
the Living with Alzheimer's Film Project

Us Against Alzheimer's

Us Against Alzheimer's

STORIES OF FAMILY, LOVE, AND FAITH

EDITED BY

Marita Golden

**WITH A FOREWORD BY DAVID SHENK
AND AN INTRODUCTION BY GEORGE VRADENBURG**

Chairman and Cofounder of UsAgainstAlzheimer's

Published in collaboration with UsAgainstAlzheimer's

Arcade Publishing • New York

First Edition

This volume includes works of fiction, in which names, places, characters, and
incidents are either the products of the author's imagination or are used fictitiously.

Arcade Publishing books may be purchased in bulk at special discounts for
sales promotion, corporate gifts, fund-raising, or educational purposes. Special
editions can also be created to specifications. For details, contact the Special Sales
Department, Arcade Publishing, 307 West 36th Street, 11th Floor, New York,
NY 10018 or arcade@skyhorsepublishing.com.

Arcade Publishing® is a registered trademark of Skyhorse Publishing, Inc.®,
a Delaware corporation.

Visit our website at www.arcadepub.com.
Visit the author's website at www.maritagolden.com.

10 9 8 7 6 5 4 3 2 1

Library of Congress Cataloging-in-Publication Data is available on file.
Library of Congress Control Number: 2019943603

Cover design by Erin Seaward-Hiatt
Cover illustration: iStockphoto

Print ISBN: 978-1-948924-14-6
Ebook ISBN: 978-1-948924-16-0

Printed in the United States of America

CONTENTS

I WON'T FORGET YOU

STRANGER THAN FICTION

FOREWORD

There's a vapid joke that so many—so, so many—people have blurted out to me over the years immediately after I mention that I'm working on a book or film or podcast about Alzheimer's: "Can you tell me again?—I've just forgotten what you're working on . . ."

If I had a nickel . . . But this ridiculous line has helped me to understand something fundamental: People *desperately* do not want to think about dementia if they don't absolutely have to.

This is our existential challenge, on top of all the awfulness of dealing directly with this disease. We have to find a way to tell everyone what they powerfully do not want to hear. We need people to understand what this disease is, in order to mitigate the loneliness, in order to build up our global infrastructure of caregiving, and in order to stop Alzheimer's once and for all.

Here is what's so beautiful about this book: It is chock full of people sticking their necks out and telling their story. With clarity, with patience, with feeling, with faith. Greg and Daisy and Cathie and Malaika and so many others. They're doing it because they have to, and because we need them to. They are the leading spears in this war. Behind them stand terrific organizations like UsAgainstAlzheimer's and Cure Alzheimer's Fund and CaringKind and TimeSlips and the Alzheimer's Association. Together, we are finally seeing a true awakening. And we know our work is just beginning.

Join us. Let us tell you our stories and then step forward to tell your own story. Be a part of the movement that will help manage this excruciating loss: the caregivers who thanklessly alter their lives to accommodate it; the artists who help us understand its depth; the activists who make noise; the writers and actors who help us convey its nuances and its toll; and the private philanthropists who dedicate their fortunes to fund unpopular research ideas.

And, of course, the scientists. Though the public cannot yet taste its fruits, there has been much progress in Alzheimer's research. We are much closer to a cure than we were a decade ago. We *will* stop this disease. In an age where our relationship to facts has suddenly become rather wobbly, we must robustly support these fact-gatherers, have faith in their methods, follow the truth wherever it takes us, and never, ever, ever give up hope.

David Shenk
Cohost of the podcast *The Forgetting:
Inside the Mind of Alzheimer's*
Author of *The Forgetting*
Creator of *The Living with Alzheimer's Film Project*

INTRODUCTION
BY GEORGE VRADENBURG

Nearly thirty years ago, my late wife's mother called at 3 a.m. to complain about a strange man in her house. We rushed over, only to find that the "strange man" was my father-in-law. By the end of her life, my wife's mother could no longer speak, move, or recognize her daughter. As with millions since, this fierce woman had been tragically swallowed up by the gaping maw of Alzheimer's.

It was experiences like this one that ultimately spurred my wife Trish and me to found UsAgainstAlzheimer's, a disruptive advocacy and research organization that has been fighting to expand treatments and accelerate toward a cure for Alzheimer's for nearly ten years. It was born out of our shared passion to beat back what is now the most devastating disease facing our population, economy, and society.

We demanded action on the Alzheimer's epidemic from senators, researchers, and the public—always with determination, grit, and, when needed, just the right touch of humor. Trish in particular had an immense gift for translating the pain and hardship associated with the disease into hopeful action—and she did it with the perfect combination of deep empathy and keen strategic thinking.

A decade later, this movement has made progress, though not enough. We have increased funding for Alzheimer's from the National Institutes of Health from $450 million to $2.4 billion; we have pressured Medicare to recognize Alzheimer's as a chronic disease on par with diabetes and hypertension; and we have had legislative successes, including the recent reintroduction of the bicameral, bipartisan CHANGE Act and the passing of the EUREKA and BOLD Acts into law. Furthermore, emerging scientific research is telling us that there are proactive, risk-reducing steps we can all take around diet, exercise, and social engagement to build resilience against cognitive decline. Despite these achievements, Alzheimer's remains the only top-ten disease in the United States without an effective treatment or cure, affecting 5.8 million diagnosed patients and 16 million caregivers at a massive cost of $290 billion annually.

These are tragic numbers, but they are statistics. For those not directly impacted, it can be easy to forget that each of those combined 21.8 million people is an individual with a story, a family, and a circumstance that is uniquely theirs. Knowing these individuals, their backgrounds, and their situations humanizes what can so easily become a generic, arm's-length conversation fraught with fear, stigma, and uncertainty. This can be even more true within communities of color, where the impact of the disease is disproportionate. (African Americans are twice as likely and Latinos are 1.5 times as likely to have Alzheimer's.)

That's why books like this one are so important, and why I was so honored to be asked to write the introduction. The work contained here brings to life personal experiences with Alzheimer's from across the world. It is real and deeply personal. It is at once heartbreaking, fearful, relatable, and funny but, most of all, human in its expression. It is a snapshot of experiences across the Alzheimer's and dementia spectrum, and offers readers—whether personally familiar with the cruelty of this disease or not—a glimpse of life for those in the midst of the struggle.

We will ultimately find a cure for this devastating disease. There's reason to be hopeful. And as organizations like UsAgainstAlzheimer's continue to fight, as individuals today continue the important work of Trish and so many others, advocating and pushing for a cure on behalf of those they know and those they don't, we must never forget the fundamentally human piece of the Alzheimer's tragedy. Work like this ensures that the individuality and uniqueness of those who have lost their identities to Alzheimer's remain in our hearts through truly courageous work.

Us Against Alzheimer's

INTRODUCTION

BY MARITA GOLDEN

The journey began with a story. A story I never expected to write. A fictional story about an African-American family impacted by Alzheimer's disease. Four years in, I discovered as part of my research the disproportionate impact of the disease on African-American families. That discovery led to another kind of story, a piece of groundbreaking journalism about why African Americans are twice as likely as whites to develop Alzheimer's and why they are so underrepresented in the clinical trials to find a cure. After the publication of the novel and the magazine story, I thought I was through. I expected Alzheimer's to let me go. To allow me to return to my normal life. But it was too late. I now knew too much about the stigma attached to the disease, and the current and looming economic, cultural, and social shifts associated with dementias. I had met too many dedicated researchers and advocates for awareness of and a meaningful societal response to a disease that is the sixth leading cause of death in America. And mostly I had met too many people living with dignity with the disease and families who found in the process of caring for their loved ones amazing grace and strength and a transformational kind of love that made all things possible. It was too late. I had become an Alzheimer's activist.

Those families, those living with Alzheimer's and other dementias, wove their way into the fabric of my life, and it is to them that I dedicate this anthology. The organization UsAgainstAlzheimer's is a leading agitator, advocate, and creator of change in the fight against Alzheimer's disease. As an African-American woman, I was deeply impressed by the organization's commitment through its out-reach networks to ensure that African Americans, women, Latinx, and other marginalized groups are at the center, seated at the table where decisions are made and questions asked that shape the public discourse and the research decisions about care and cures.

Alzheimer's is an irreversible, progressive brain disorder that slowly destroys memory and thinking skills and eventually the ability to carry out simple tasks. Five and a half million Americans have Alzheimer's disease. There is no cure. Alzheimer's is the most common form of dementia, of which there are numerous types; all of them affect mental cognition.

George Vradenburg founded UsAgainstAlzheimer's with his late wife, Trish.

George is a visionary, a man with a mission, a genius at inspiring action and making change happen. In its nine years of existence the organization has had global impact. I am a child of the sixties—activism is in my DNA—so when I couldn't forget those families and those individuals living with dementias, I knew I had received my next assignment. Writing for me is an act of dialogue not just with my imagination but with readers, society, and my own soul. If I can't give a reader a new way to see the world, why write? And that is how this anthology, *Us Against Alzheimer's: Stories of Family, Love, and Faith*, was born. All the royalties from this anthology will go to support the work of UsAgainstAlzheimer's.

I have learned much of what I know about Alzheimer's disease from Dr. Goldie Byrd, director of the Maya Angelou Center for Health Disparities at Wake Forest University, as well as Stephanie Monroe and Jason Resendez of UsAgainstAlzheimer's and John Dwyer of the Global Alzheimer's Platform. They are among the army of dedicated people serving on the front lines in the fight against this disease.

My goal with this project was simple yet ambitious: to capture in nonfiction and fiction narratives the wrenching experience of watching a loved one consumed by a disease that essentially kills them twice. Once as they forget who they are and then when their bodies succumb to the full-blown effects of dementia. But I mostly wanted to provide readers with a peek into what I had discovered in five years of research, that this cruel disease is as much about the spirit and heart of those it afflicts and their families as it is about brain cells.

Again and again, I was buoyed by the testimony of siblings, parents, and others who stood by and stood up for those with Alzheimer's and were blessed by the experience. Blessed in the midst of sleepless nights and self-doubt and anger and grief. I'll never forget the words of a young man on a panel at one of the annual UsAgainstAlzheimer's conferences, describing how it felt, and how enlarged he had been by caring for his mother who in her mid-sixties was being claimed by dementia day by day. He spoke of having to give up his full-time job but also of tender moments and revelations and things said he had never expected. He told the audience, "I tell my siblings who leave most of the care of our mother to me, 'You should come and get some of this. Before it's too late.'"

I am extremely proud of this project. I am proud of the immense generosity of the writers who eagerly donated their stories once I told them about UsAgainstAlzheimer's. I am proud also that this is a multicultural collection. Alzheimer's is a disease with global impact. The stories on these pages represent the experiences of writers from all over the US and from India, Trinidad, Haiti, and the Dominican Republic. The contributors are award-winning published authors, caregivers turned writers, Alzheimer's activists, and those living with Alzheimer's.

This collection is divided into four sections, three of which represent the various seasons of the Alzheimer's experience. In "Turning Points," you'll read accounts of the gradual realization of the immensity of dementia's impact on families and relationships. How do you find your way through the dark and murky waters of denial and land on the shore of acceptance? How do you let go of the hope for a different reality and accept that there is no turning back, only more turning points? When are you prepared to ask for help, for yourself as one with the disease or as caregiver? How can you, how do you decide that assisted living or a dementia care unit is the only viable option?

How do you move past guilt? These are the decisions that mark new chapters in an unfolding, confounding story.

In "All That Remains," the narratives address the discovery that the person with Alzheimer's is more than the disease. Their world is one that has to be accepted and entered. All that remains is often much more than could be expected. To see *all* that remains requires a vision shaped by respect and love and the ability to live on Planet Alzheimer's, to learn new rules and a new language.

In "I Won't Forget You," writers consider the legacy left by a parent, spouse, or friend and come to both a reckoning with and a recognition of Alzheimer's as a symbol of long-standing absences, amnesia, distance, and forgetting. A symbol of the resilience of loyalty and unbroken bonds. A symbol of the fact that there is no forgetting, for there is always life after death in our hearts.

In the "Fiction" section, the narratives mine the pathos, terror, and even the humor (and, yes, there can be humor) in how Alzheimer's disease takes shape and finds expression. Fiction, with its requirement to suspend disbelief, may be the most natural home for meditations on the Alzheimer's experience. The subject of all the stories in this section, however, is not disease or death, but the meaning of life.

It is my hope that you will find in this book a deeper understanding of the courage of families impacted by Alzheimer's and other dementias. I hope you are lifted and renewed by their daily witness to family, love, and faith.

TURNING POINTS

INTRODUCTION

There is no one turning point for those living with dementia, for family members, caretakers, or friends. The disease evolves like an unhinged, intemperate, willful dance. A dance whose steps are ever changing. A dance that leaves those performing it breathless. The turning points are those spaces and those places where instinct and understanding unfold quietly amid the din, and an anointing somehow takes place. There is no going back, because you stand shocked and grateful that this place that promises only what is here and now feels like home. The narratives in this section capture the mysterious ways that turning points arrive and impose a "new world order" on the whirlwind and drama of dementia and Alzheimer's.

There is the turning to face the big picture that is embedded in visits to the doctor, medications, exhaustion, tried patience, blank stares, and the gradual inching away of memory. Where else would the big picture be if not seeded in the soil of the mundane? There is the turning to face the emotional truth that meaning springs from the ordinary. We take, and hold in our bodies and our hands, responsibility for another and for ourselves. We love the broken body and mind because we see in it the outline of our own looming fragility.

And if we have made our own luck, by standing still and tall and standing up to the disease, by morphing into witness and not just friend or family, but witness as in "can I *get* a witness" for my trials and trouble and pain, there is the turning into a person who finally knows what is happening, what this disease teaches us about the deeper promises of life lived and honored in its terrible moments of reckoning.

ALZHEIMER'S AND THE ER
JANE BANDLER

I received a call at 8:00 a.m. from the director of the assisted living community where my husband, Don, had been living for the past year and a half. It was a small facility, and Don was one of the most active and loved residents. He was physically strong and upbeat. He enjoyed participating in all activities, greeted everyone, and walked around as if he was the ambassador of the place. This was how Don was before he had Alzheimer's too. I thought the day my children and I brought him to the assisted living was the worst day of my life. But that was before I had adopted the philosophy that each *today* was going to be the best day an Alzheimer's patient or caregiver was going to have because the *future* did not hold any hope.

On that early morning call, the director told me that Don was extremely angry and agitated. His behavior was aggressive and, as a result, they had determined that he had to be sent to the emergency room of a nearby hospital. I said I didn't understand why that was necessary and I would prefer they waited until I got there. I had heard many horror stories about what happens to Alzheimer's patients at the hospital. Back in 1996 when my mother had Alzheimer's, my father and I received a call from her assisted living that we should go directly to the hospital, and the memory of that came flooding into my mind.

Anxious and very afraid, I jumped into my car and drove the twenty-five miles I had driven almost every day for the past eighteen months. I felt reassured that they would not send Don to the hospital until I got there and I could accompany him if necessary. Mid-drive, my cell phone rang, and I heard the strained voice of the director asking when I would arrive. I told her I was almost there. When I did arrive and walked into the familiar reception area, the directors and staff were standing by the front door waiting for me. I could feel the tension. They told me Don was already at the emergency room. They simply could not wait for me as his behavior had become too violent. They said they wanted me to come to the assisted living first so they could tell me face to face how out of control Don had become. They were traumatized themselves and wanted to be sure I was prepared for what I was going to see at the hospital. Don was dangerously out of control, and for the safety of the other residents, they had had no choice but to call the police to escort him in an ambulance to the hospital. They hoped the hospital would be able to medicate him and calm him down. Now I was even more worried, and I felt angry that I hadn't been notified much earlier. I felt I could have been there for Don at his darkest moments. I didn't understand what had happened. But in my nine years of caregiving for Don, I had learned that I had to put one foot in front of the other and face each obstacle as it came. So I followed my instinct, got in the car, and just hoped I would somehow get to the hospital. I had never been to this hospital, and I wasn't able to focus on the verbal directions the staff gave me. I had hoped one of them would accompany me and help me at this critical and scary moment, but they said they could not go with me. Of course, I found my way. And it was even more upsetting than I had imagined.

As soon as the emergency room doors opened, I could hear my husband, a French Legion of Honor recipient, a lifelong diplomat with the US State Department, and a former ambassador to Cyprus, screaming vile obscenities at the top of his lungs. I was shocked to see that there were both police and hospital security stationed outside his room. I walked up to the door to Don's room and said, "I'm his wife, what's going on?" One of the security guards said he did not think I should go in the room as my husband was violent and they were trying to get him under control. The guards told me Don was speaking nonsense, which they called "word salad." I nervously asked questions but could not concentrate when they answered because of the barrage of violent and ugly swear words Don was screaming and shouting. How was he finding these words, I wondered, as very little recognizable language had come out of his mouth in months?

I said I would like to go in, and they again advised against it. I knew I had to help Don. Since his diagnosis of early onset Alzheimer's, I'd been the only one who could console him. He could no longer speak for himself. He could not advocate for himself. He must have been crazed with fear, and I now know he was incapable of making his brain pull back from his aggressive behavior.

It was as if the hospital staff was unaware that Don had Alzheimer's, even though he had been picked up in an ambulance from a memory care assisted living facility. When I opened the door with my shaking hands, I saw my naked husband handcuffed to an ER bed, writhing and screaming, held down by six strong police officers and security guards. I didn't look at them. I looked at my husband. I wanted my voice to sound strong for him, so I willed myself to hold back my tears and fear. Don was a big, strong, six-foot-one, two hundred-pound man, and despite his mind being consumed by Alzheimer's, his body had remained strong. He was only sixty-nine years old, having been diagnosed with early onset Alzheimer's at the age of sixty-one.

When I walked in, Don didn't see me. He was too caught up in his fear, anger, and screaming, and the guards' attempts to put him in hand and leg restraints so they could remove the handcuffs that kept him in the bed only seemed to outrage him more. I walked the length of the room, squeezing behind several of the security guards, and went right up to my husband's face. I have no idea what words I said. But Don stopped mid-scream and turned his head to look at me. He immediately relaxed his tense body and silently collapsed. I started to stroke his arm and reassure him and tell him that I wasn't going anywhere. My voice soothed his exhausted mind and body. After a few minutes, I exchanged a quick glance with the one female police officer. She then quietly told the other five security guards to back off and give us space. The officers released Don and stepped back. He lay limp, looking at me in relief. A few minutes later all the guards left the room and it was just me, Don, and the ER nurse.

It was then that I knew I was Don's caregiver, his security, and that our bond of love could not be broken. I was the one who knew him better than anyone else in the world. I was the one who had to guide him through the rest of his life because Alzheimer's disease had destroyed his beautiful mind. Throughout this nine-year battle, my husband's heart and soul were still very much intact, and his love for me and trust that I would be there for him never faltered. From such an ugly and unfortunate situation, I was able to feel his love and trust. I will forever carry with me the feeling that Alzheimer's took almost everything from him but not our love for each other.

The hospital ER nurse told me I was his hero. The police officers came back to the hospital two days later to check on Don and to tell me that they had never seen anything like the reaction Don had when I arrived. They wanted to personally apologize to me that I had to see my husband being restrained like that.

I appreciated their words and their care, and it always made me proud when people acknowledged my caregiving role. But what I really wanted from them was an apology for what appeared to be their lack of knowledge and understanding that Don had Alzheimer's disease. For not seeing or feeling that he was scared out of his mind, felt physically and mentally threatened, and needed reassuring. I wanted them to apologize for not treating him with the dignity and kindness he needed and deserved. I wanted them to apologize for the fact that hospital staff and police officers are not trained to see and understand someone with Alzheimer's, a disease affecting millions of people and the sixth leading cause of death in the USA.

Sadly, my love story ended in the same hospital setting I had walked into several weeks earlier. Don spent three weeks in that hospital because he was labeled violent and none of the geriatric psychiatric hospitals would accept him. It took three weeks of constant phone calls and research before Don got transferred to a psychiatric hospital. It was there that I hoped they could adjust his medications to help his demented brain and his behavior.

But it was too late. In those three weeks, Don forgot how to walk and lost his will to live. One day, Don sat up and looked me straight in the eye and said the only clear sentence I had heard in months. "Jane, I can't do this anymore."

As a family, we followed my husband's wishes and his lead, and within a week he was transferred to hospice care in Rockville. Don refused food and water and died peacefully, surrounded by his two daughters, his son, and me, on February 24, 2017, at the age of sixty-nine.

EVERY 68 SECONDS

An Excerpt from *Slow Dancing with a Stranger:
Lost and Found in the Age of Alzheimer's*

MERYL COMER

The man I live with is not the man I fell in love with and married.

He has slowly been robbed of something we all take for granted: the ability to navigate the mundane activities of daily living—bathing, shaving, dressing, feeding, and using the bathroom. His inner clock is confused and can't be reset. His eyes are vacant and unaware—as if an internal window shade veils our access.

Before I grasped what was happening, I was hurt and annoyed by my husband's behavior. Those feelings dissolved into unconditional empathy once I understood the cruelty of his diagnosis: early-onset Alzheimer's disease. He was fifty-eight.

At first, I ran interference and fought for him because it was the right thing to do. He was slipping out of control—confused, childlike, and helpless, his social filters stripped away. He shadowed me because I was familiar and safe, even when he could no longer remember my name.

I always loved him, but during our marriage, he was often aloof and unreachable. In illness, unlike in health, he made me feel needed and important to him.

Neither a scientist nor neurologist, I have spent close to two decades trying to decipher what's going on in my husband's head. How hard and unfair it is for such a smart man to lose pieces of his intellect and independence as the circuitry of his brain misfires and corrodes. No new short-term memories stick: his internal navigational compass has shut down. His disease is my crossword puzzle.

Harvey has long forgotten me, but I am constant as his copilot and guardian. Every conversation is inclusive and respectful even though he is often unintelligible or mute. It is a charade that never ends. I bear the burden of all decisions for us both. The demons and terror of his world define mine. Any challenge is self-defeating. I play into his reality and pretend that his fate and our life together are not doomed. Unfortunately, I know better.

Alzheimer's distorts and destroys shared memories that bind family ties. Caregivers are not unlike victims who survive a hurricane and find ourselves sifting through the rubble to rescue faded, storm-drenched photos or sentimental objects. We piece together what's left of our past and struggle to put down building blocks for the future. I need to make some sense of my journey through this storm.

My bookshelf is lined with tomes on dementia care, yet the page I need always seems to be missing. Each brain unravels in its own quirky and idiosyncratic way. I have learned firsthand that there is no single solution to taking care of someone with dementia.

Many times, personal stories involving Alzheimer's gloss over the unseemly details of care. They are written as love stories of unquestioned devotion or living memorials to honor someone during better times. Why not? As spouses and caregivers, we deserve to do whatever works for us. It is our version of pain management. But I never wanted to embellish or soften the edges around the truth. It does not do justice to the cruelty of the disease. I offer you my own experiences from a position of hard-won humility. I hope you will thread them with your own.

When I say I have cared full-time for Harvey in our home all these years, many ask me why. Even now, there is always an initial reflex that makes me want to say, "Do I really need to explain myself after all I've been through?"

I realize that the question is a natural one, a human one, a social one. The interlocutors are not judging me, but rather vicariously checking themselves. In questioning me, they are testing their own capacity to deal with a diagnosis of Alzheimer's disease and the potential impact it might have on their relationship with a partner or parent.

When people hear my story, they sometimes tell me they wouldn't make the same choices. I do not hold myself up as an example to follow. No one who has been on the frontlines of care ever questions when someone says "I can't do this anymore." But I do want to be part of the last generation of caregivers trapped by a loved one's diagnosis, and a troublesome lack of quality care options.

When it comes to Alzheimer's, caregivers are frequently too worn out or isolated to protest. Perhaps this is why advocacy around the disease has often lacked the passion and energy that characterize the cancer and HIV communities. But how will people understand if we do not tell our stories without apology?

Alzheimer's disease today affects a reported 5.4 million people in the United States and 44 million worldwide. Like a stealth invader, it is quietly dementing aging populations globally all while quickly pushing past cancer and HIV/AIDS as the most critical public health problem of our time. Every sixty-eight seconds, another one of us falls victim. Yet, 50 percent of those with dementia never get diagnosed.

My greatest fear is that mine will be the family next door by mid-century.

There is not a single FDA-approved drug that actually slows the progression of Alzheimer's disease. There have been too many failed late-stage clinical trials with promising drugs that seemed to work—until it became clear that they did not.

Sometimes I think we would be better off if Alzheimer's disease was a brand-new emergency instead of a century-old threat to which we somehow have become inured. Perhaps people would understand that when it comes to disease, everyone is a stakeholder, because everyone is at risk.

There are also fifteen million caregivers just like me; unintended victims and not among the official count. Add to our legions those caring for loved ones—young and old—with diseases of the brain, traumatic brain injuries, and other chronic diseases complicated by a memory disorder. We speak the same language. Our numbers amplify the collective pain that makes it impossible for me to rest.

The only way to minimize the effects of Alzheimer's disease is to get out in front of it; delay its onset or even reverse its devastation of the mind. We need to move toward early diagnosis and study adults who do not yet show symptoms. People like you and me.

Such a decision entails hard personal choices, risks, and emotional discomfort. It means demanding safe and clinically valid genetic tests that let us learn if we are at higher risk for getting Alzheimer's disease. It requires managing our lives and choices under the shadow of the possibility of disease.

Those of us who are fifty years and older must stop viewing ourselves as ageless. All of us should track our cognitive health, just as we do cholesterol levels or blood pressure. We need to overcome fear and stop cowering in the shadows of stigma.

I write for all of us who are still well, but have seen the devastation of Alzheimer's disease firsthand. The emergency is with us and in us.

I write to clinicians, reluctant to diagnose because they can't effectively treat. Please know the inadvertent trauma you inflict on families left confused, hurt, and helpless. Then time runs out on the ultimate conversation with our loved ones about end-of-life wishes. Their minds are erased. It is simply too late.

I write to reach the generation of our adult sons and daughters, who struggle to understand our loves as we care for a loved one with Alzheimer's. They stand on the precipice and wrestle with issues and decisions similar to the ones we have faced. They deserve better options and not the bankrupting burden of our care. This is not the legacy we want for our children or the way anyone wishes to be remembered.

I write for my grandchildren because, no matter how hard I tried, Alzheimer's blanketed my home with sadness. I know that loving each of them unconditionally has been my salvation. One day, I hope they read these words and appreciate my choices.

As I write these words, a faint glow fills the room I share with Harvey. He is always present, even though he is absent. There is an intimacy in our isolation.

ME FE NOS SOSTIENE (MY FAITH SUSTAINS US)

Daisy Duarte,
as told to Lynda Everman and Don Wendorf

I say that my faith sustains "us" instead of "me" because I am now taking care of my mom, who has advanced Alzheimer's disease. Mom raised my brother and sister and me in the suburbs of Chicago, mostly by herself and in spite of several tough, even abusive relationships. I was the "troublemaker" kid who really gave her a run for her money. Mom got up at 4:00 a.m. each morning and rode four buses and one train to work in the inner city as a teacher's aide, regardless of the sometimes harsh Chicago weather. These were often difficult times, but she taught us to have faith: "*Dios prevalecerá, tu saldrás bien.*" God will prevail; you'll come out of it. It may take years, she said, but you will.

Mom was a devout churchgoer, and she taught us to love the church. We were baptized as Catholics, although Mom eventually found a nondenominational Bible church she loved. She went to church every Wednesday and Friday night and again on Sunday and even found time to cook on Saturdays for homeless people. She loved the practical life lessons she heard at church and felt the Lord was "speaking right to her."

My brother left for the Marines at seventeen, and when my sister was about seventeen, she had a baby and moved to Missouri. Mom and I stayed in Chicago for a time, and then I moved to Missouri to work in my sister's and brother-in-law's restaurant. When I was in my early thirties, I opened my own sports bar, which I loved. But when Mom was about fifty-five years old, she started getting sick and showing lots of problems with memory and her emotions. We moved Mom to Missouri, and I became Mom's caregiver in my home.

Mom was misdiagnosed at first, and we had some very tough times. For a while, she was able to help some at my sports bar, but at one point she told my then thirteen-year-old nephew to stab her with one of the kitchen knives, even though she had seemed her usual happy, social self. I closed the sports bar and took her home, where the next morning she was still crying and screaming, "God, stop telling me to kill myself." She was hallucinating, and I took her to the hospital, where they stopped all her medications, which actually helped a little. After a lot more testing, they concluded she had Creutzfeldt-Jakob disease and would die within six to nine months. I took her home, intending to take care of her there until she died. I promised Mom I would never put her in an institution. That was eight years ago.

I did a lot of research, found new doctors, and new tests finally revealed the diagnosis of Alzheimer's disease. I had had to close down my business, and for the next three years I was her full-time caregiver at home. I didn't have any social life and suffered some depression but was glad Mom and I could share a lot together, including the Christian music we both loved so much.

I never questioned becoming Mom's caregiver, even when it cost me a romantic relationship when my partner at that time insisted Mom needed to be put in a home. But my faith and the values of the Hispanic community of taking care of our parents ourselves at home made my decision clear. They did it for us; we have to do it for them. Mom taught us to be independent and to be fighters. My love for her and the help of the Lord keep me going. The only two people I can thank my whole life from the bottom of my heart are my mom and the Lord.

Every morning I start our day by kissing Mom and putting my hand on her head as I make the sign of the cross on her forehead with my thumb. I pray for us by saying, "Thank you, Lord, for giving us another day of life" and "Thank you for dying on the cross for our sins. Forgive us for any of our sins and may you guide us through our day." Then we do the morning routine of changing diapers, getting cleaned up, feeding her breakfast, getting dressed, combing her hair, and brushing her tongue. On days I work, she is taken care of by my nephew and my partner, who put her to bed days I work late at my brother-in-law's restaurant.

Even if Mom is asleep when I get home, we end the day with the sign of the cross again and a talking prayer about how the day went. Then I pray for us and thank God for another day and for guiding us through it. I add that "whenever you need to give Mom her wings, I know she's ready" if that is His will.

In the process of finding the right diagnosis for Mom, I learned from her family in Puerto Rico that nearly 75 percent of Mom's family has suffered from Alzheimer's going back for generations. As a result of learning this, I enrolled in the Dominantly Inherited Alzheimer's Network research study at the Washington University School of Medicine in St. Louis and learned in 2015 that I tested positive for the early-onset familial Alzheimer's gene.

That means that I will probably have the disease by my sixty-fifth birthday. I am now in my early forties, living with the knowledge that my memories have a limited shelf life, set to expire in twenty-five years. This was all gut-wrenching to go through, and I cried when I first heard my diagnosis. But I want to be able to help my Mom and the rest of the family and the community.

I decided to use my time to fight for a cure as an advocate, a caregiver, and as one of the few Latina participants in an Alzheimer's clinical trial. Latinos are 1.5 times more at risk for Alzheimer's, and more than 1.8 million Latino family members care for an individual with dementia. Most are daughters like me who believe in taking care of our loved ones ourselves. I also became a spokesperson for LatinosAgainstAlzheimer's and I lobby for Congress to give more funds for research.

Caregiving is a high-stress, around-the-clock job. Often the ones we care for don't remember who we are and cannot dress, feed, or bathe themselves. It takes love, a sense of duty and honor, and lots of help from others. But, my mom taught me: "*Si tienes amor sin condiciones, tú puedes emprender todo.*" If you have unconditional love, you can tackle anything. She always told us: "*Dios prevalecerá, tu saldrás bien.*" God will prevail; you'll come out of it. I believe in my mom and in the Word of the Lord. My faith sustains us.

THE WAY IN
Marita Golden

The first time I sat in a group of men and women diagnosed with Alzheimer's disease I felt fear. I have, as I write this, traveled so far from that emotion, that response, that I say the words without any shame. It wasn't anxiety or nervousness that had my heart beating a bit faster, although what I felt was surely related to the kind of uncertainty produced by those responses. No, I felt fear. **Shameless admission number one.** The men and women, whose average age was in the middle seventies, were residents of the memory care unit in an assisted living residence where I was doing research for a novel about an African-American family dealing with the impact of Alzheimer's disease. I was sitting in on a late morning session with the residents, listening to their stories, remembrances, and memories prompted by gentle questioning from a certified nursing assistant. The session was designed to stimulate memories essentially of who these men and women used to be. The question was: "Tell us about the work you used to do."

The fear I felt was, I now know, like most fear, irrational, ego-driven, and largely based on hypothetical what-ifs. It seems that we humans are always performing and always expecting others to perform for us. So some of the fear I know was inspired by the expectation that this group of mostly calm and gentle, well-dressed seniors would *do something, say something, be someone* that my arsenal of responses and reactions had not prepared me to handle. There was also the expectation that I, in the midst of a group of people labeled as diminished and intellectually incapacitated, *would do something, say something, be someone* at odds with the vision of myself as capable and in control of most situations.

Then there was the other fear, the one that haunted me as I spent hours among these people who had lived lives of career and material success that allowed them to be cared for in a residence that did not accept Medicare and cost $5,000.00 a month. The fear that was raw and chilling in the early days of my research, the fear that Alzheimer's would, as it had come for them, come for me.

But perhaps the deepest and most awful fear was that these men and women were lacking, because of Alzheimer's, a core, an essence, that would allow me to touch them and to be touched by them, to hear and see them for who they had been and, more importantly, who they were now. I knew I could not write a novel about Alzheimer's if I could not imagine myself as living and breathing inside their skin.

During the four years I spent researching the novel, I did not "get over" fear as much as I allowed the vibrant, life-giving wisdom and humanity of these men and women to chip away at and dismantle it. And that happened because I was willing to hear and then to listen. What I heard and listened to wove a connecting thread between me and people I was "studying" at first and then came to recognize as my shadow, my echo in ways that had nothing at all to do with Alzheimer's disease.

From that day I remember the tall, clean-shaven man who sat in the group, legs crossed, periodically shifting his baseball cap on his nearly bald head as he smiled with proud satisfaction and told us, "I worked for the Treasury Department and kept our money safe." The description of his job sounds so elementary, almost childlike, and yet isn't that what the Treasury Department does? Keep the nation's money safe?

The plump, copper-colored woman whose cheeks were smeared with rouge and whose gray curls were topped by a felt hat told us that she had been a teacher. In response to questioning, she could not recall what grade she taught or the name of her school. But I watched her eyes sparkle in the moments before she closed them tightly and for fifteen minutes twice recited a poem her students had to memorize.

For most of human history, poems enabled the passing of stories between generations—think of *The Iliad* or Langston Hughes's "The Negro Speaks of Rivers." Poems capture moments and experiences in a new way and communicate one soul to another. Listening to a poem whose title was no longer remembered, watching the fervor with which it was recited, I knew how much that woman's students had meant to her, and how for her teaching was more art than science. That poem was a fragmentary memory of her whole life.

And there was also the agitated woman sitting beside me, who during breaks in the session responded to my smile with a stream of rambling, repetitive fragments about being a student at Hampton University. Her eyes were both ablaze with life and somehow shell-shocked as she repeated over and over that she lived on campus and had joined the AKA sorority. Clearly, the sisterhood, the sense of mission, the bonds that are the glue inspiring loyalty among sorors gave as much meaning to that woman's life as she sat beside me as it had maybe fifty years earlier.

That day I learned that Alzheimer's does not rob us of memories as much as it shifts them around in the house we call our mind. Some get stored in the attic and are rarely touched; others once consigned to the basement are retrieved and given a place of dominance and pride. As I read more about the disease, I came to understand that it is when one can no longer remember, recall, or even learn anything (as a result of the gradual failure of the brain to activate and spur the body to function) that the disease becomes fatal. The absence of memories kills us. We die without the ability to recall who we had been, who we are. What, I wondered, would I remember? What, in the midst of encroaching death, would stubbornly give me life?

* * *

I should have expected the request. In fact, I would have been surprised if at some point it had not come. Still, when it came, my reflexive tendency to overthink and over-plan and over-worry immediately took me hostage. The director of the facility asked me to do a reading and discussion of my work for the residents. Musicians, artists, journalists, she told me, had been guest speakers as part of a program designed to keep the residents connected to the world outside of the facility as well as intellectually stimulated. I knew that I would say yes, and I did, without hesitation even as I wondered if the months I had spent embedded in the lives of the residents, sitting in on their exercises, eating lunch with them in the cafeteria, talking to the certified nursing assistants who cared for them, would not somehow be compromised if I shifted gears. But of course, there was something more. **Shameless admission number two:** I agreed to do a reading, yet wondered what a reading would mean for *me*? How would my writer's ego be fed by an audience that might not comprehend everything I was saying? What if they asked a question I could not answer? Oddly, I never worried about that with other audiences. This phalanx of largely trivial concerns was continuing evidence of how far I still had to go before I was wedded to these men and women, before I saw them as my brother/sister from another mother, as people who I did not have to strive to understand because, although I still did not fully know it, I understood them already because I understood myself.

A digressive note here about understanding oneself and freewill, independence, and control. Since completing the novel, I have read more and more about how as humans we live both burdened and fueled by the belief that free will, independence, and control are the engines of our existence. In reality we are animals activated and controlled mostly by brain synapses, hormones, and genes. Sex, hunger, ambition, creativity, love, fear . . . it may all be a bundle of urges that positions us in a grueling lifelong position of subservience to the whims of our internal biology and architecture.

But as I prepared for my reading, I wasn't aware of that. I still thought that the best plan was to have a plan, even with an audience of people forced to improvise each moment. I had to have a plan. I had to know what to expect. I had to know what might happen.

Sitting before the residents that afternoon, I had a plan. I had scrapped my original plan, which was to read from one of my novels and then take questions. By now I knew that my audiences' attention span was more hope than reality, that in fact I had at best about twenty minutes to engage and depart, and that rather than a sumptuous several-course meal, I would make my offering in the equivalent of appetizers.

I took a deep breath, one I hoped no one could hear, and began by saying, "I'm a writer, and I grew up here in Washington, DC. Writing has taken me all over the world." Then rather than talking about my writing process and the subjects I chose, I shared how satisfying, wondrous, and wonderful it had been to have been given a gift that I honored and that became the vehicle for my discovery of so many other countries and people.

I shared the experience of traveling to Jamaica to write a travel article and sitting on the beaches on Negril, of serving as an "official" writer representing the United States in Turkey on a cultural visit to that country, of attending a writer's conference in London. The name of each city or country inspired someone in the audience to call out, "I've been there"; "That was where we had our honeymoon"; "I went there for vacation." Memory and memories inspired residents to eagerly raise their hands seeking my recognition or simply to stand and claim their storytelling space. What they shared were mostly heartfelt fragments of the joy of discovering a new land, a new people, and in the process a new self. Now I sat back and listened. For listening and observing, hearing and seeing are the foundations of writing. Words only get on the page because I have listened to my heart or someone else's, and because imagination introduces me, like faith, to the power and reality of the unseen and the unknown. So, allowing the residents to tell me their stories of the borders they had crossed was part of my continuing education. I thought I had come to tell them stories, but they forged an environment where we told stories to one another. And so, this reading was no different than any other.

And then a resident recalled visiting Paris and blushed as she said, "I was there in April with someone I loved." The room shuddered with appreciative laughter. There is much that those with Alzheimer's "forget," but there is so much more that they remember—love, desire, friendship, hope, dreams. I was no longer steering our craft and took another deep breath, this time one that signaled my surrender to go wherever we were headed. A frayed but beautiful tapestry was woven in the next few minutes from silence I did not rush to fill, and more fragments, rough-hewn jewels of people and places were tossed into our midst.

Then I reached for the book I had brought: my novel *Long Distance Life*, about sixty years in the life of a family headed by a woman who migrates from Spring Hope, North Carolina, to Washington, DC, in the 1930s as part of the great migration of African Americans from the South. The book was inspired by my mother's life, yet was a vastly different story. I had chosen a paragraph to read, and in the quiet moments after the last word, the woman who had been in Paris with someone she loved stood up and pointed to me in what I initially thought was an accusatory stance, and shouted, "I know that woman."

Those are the words that every writer longs to hear from a listener or a reader, "I know that story, I know that woman, that man, that child." And we understand that then we have done our job, for what is *known* is known literally, or spiritually, or metaphorically and sometimes all three. And that is what the woman whose name I later learned was Gladys meant. She knew the character in the novel and would in some sense take her with her when she left the small den where we sat.

When Gladys announced, "I know that woman," I felt, in a long-awaited moment of anointing, that I finally knew her and the other women and men in the room with us. I began to feel that I could write this story.

* * *

So now I knew I could create and imagine this story, but how would I actually do it? What would that mean, look, and feel like for me and for my characters? Although I consider *The Wide Circumference of Love* largely a story of how married love and self-love are transformed by a wrenching crisis, it is grounded in the experience of one man, Gregory Tate, experiencing and living with Alzheimer's disease. The novel opens on the day that Gregory's wife, Diane, takes him to live in a memory care unit because he has been diagnosed with early-onset Alzheimer's. It is the story of their thirty-five-year marriage and their prodigal son and dutiful daughter.

I relied on several "experts," who read various drafts and helped me accurately portray the disease and how it manifested in the body and mind of those with it, as well as its impact on family members, friends, and caregivers. The experts included the wife of a resident of the memory care unit I spent time at and a social worker on staff at the center as well as a senior health consultant who helped families caring for those with Alzheimer's disease.

Although often the actions of those with Alzheimer's and other dementias appear "crazy," these individuals have not lost their minds. The writing challenge was to dramatize both the strangeness of actions induced by the diminishment of cognitive abilities and simultaneously capture the ways that what these individuals still possessed bound them to us.

After reading an early draft in which I was attempting to write from the point of view of Gregory, the staff social worker informed me gently that I still had work to do. "Remember," she said, "when writing about a person with this disease, nothing that you can imagine is off limits, no matter how odd, incongruous or inexplicable." My descriptions of Gregory, she told me, were too safe and lacked the edge and tension built into the experience of Alzheimer's. The kind of tension and edge that for a long time I had feared and that had erected a wall between me and the residents.

She then told me about the resident who had been a farmer and who often urinated in the potted plants in the hallway because he imagined himself watering his crops and the retired fireman who, each time he heard a loud noise, thought it was a fire alarm and banged on residents' doors trying to evacuate them from the building.

Ultimately, I wrote a scene that captured Gregory's vulnerability, his fear as well as his all-too-natural and recognizable yearning to feel a sense of control. It is a scene early in his acclimation to living in the residence. It is midnight, and he is walking the halls naked. Naked because he is not only stripped of clothing but also of inhibition and the self he once knew, the self he once was. He is naked walking the halls fleeing he knows not what, but searching for a way out of this place and back to himself. He wants to go home, and *home* is who he used to be. In the midst of a near scuffle with a nursing assistant who wants to guide him back to his room, another resident, a woman who has fallen in love with him, opens her door and offers a sheet to cover his body. As anyone in love would do, she offers protection.

The writing of that scene was possible because I mined my own generalized, ever-present vulnerabilities and used them as a springboard into the experience of a sixty-nine-year-old former architect with Alzheimer's. A man who was a father, husband, friend, brother, son, builder, and who remained all those things in the midst of the most massive upheaval he has ever known.

* * *

How did I find myself in this place? No one in my family had Alzheimer's, and it is a topic that I previously had little interest in. Yet writing a novel about Alzheimer's was as understandable as other topics I had explored in fiction, among them the death of a child and the work and commitment of civil rights activists. I had known very little about either of those subjects before the novels I wrote inspired by them plunged me into a world of imagination that literally possessed me in each case for several years.

I am drawn to write about what I don't know, and when I write about what I in theory "know," I still write to discover what I don't. There is a word for that: inspiration. But for me a more precise designation is that I have been "called." Being called means finding answers as well as being swept away by a tidal wave of questions. Questions for my characters and questions for me. Fiction creates imagined lives and invades my own.

Watching families wrestle and live with the burdens, challenges, and sometimes gifts of Alzheimer's disease flooded me with questions. Who would care for me? What kind of caregiver would I be? These are not questions answered easily, or only once. And, like many questions, they have more than one answer.

I set out to write not an Alzheimer's story but a love story, and I did. Now I know what the individuals who opened their lives to me know: that love, the kind that can withstand the onslaught of this disease and even blossom in its harsh, glaring light, is stubborn, persistent, resilient, impatient, and sometimes confused, and it never walks away.

FATHER FIGURES
Evans D. Hopkins

Seven years after my release from prison, I was living a very full life, writing a memoir and caring for my elderly parents, Daniel and Marguerite Hopkins. I would write well into the night, as had become my custom during my years of incarceration. On this summer night, I had the phone ringer off so I could get into the groove. I happened to take a break around 3 a.m., to gauge whether I could push it for another hour, and it was then that I caught a glimpse of the blinking red light on the base unit of my portable phone.

I checked the message, and it was Anita, my parents' caregiver, her voice full of alarm.

"Derrell, you need to come out here quick. Your father has had a stroke or something. Call or come right away."

I was into my car in five minutes, glad that I was still up and dressed as I raced beneath the city streetlamps of Danville, Virginia, sixty and seventy miles per hour, then hitting eighty or ninety once I reached the county line. I prayed that Pop was still alive, that this was just an ordinary alarm, something that medicine—and I, psychologi-cally—could handle. Then I thought of the irony of my prayer: how, during such episodes, even the most hardened man will return to his roots, to prayer, as if one's prayers might influence how the cells and fluids within our aged loved ones' bodies will react, as if our thoughts might influence their illnesses.

The scene at the house in rural Pittsylvania County was fraught with alarm, red lights from the volunteer rescue squad's ambulance and gigantic SUV flashing off the great pines bordering the property.

I drove past them onto the lawn, crazily thinking of how I was damaging the grass.

Upon entering the house, I was met by one of the five attendants, all of them white. "You remember me, don't you?" one of them said, in his farm-boy drawl, eager that I might recognize him. "Your father lets me hunt out here," he rambled on, and rather than being irritated, I could not help thinking kindly of the white boy, wanting me to know that he was a good guy, trying to give the extra effort, to show some personal appreciation to the family.

"I sure do," I lied, as he led me to the bedroom, where Anita was helping Pop into his jacket. The other attendants hovered over him, and Mama, who had become ever more silent, in the grip of fairly advanced Parkinson's disease, sat quietly on the opposite side of the bed. "It seems like he's had a stroke or something," the lone woman attendant said. The older male who seemed to be in charge took over then, telling me that they weren't sure if my father was normally as weak and spacey as he seemed, or if this was his normal state.

"His vital signs seem to be all right, but he doesn't seem to know where he is," he said. I noticed right away that Pop's mouth seemed to be turned down slightly—not a good sign—but I was nearly jubilant with relief that he was sitting up, not stretched out in the throes of a seizure or some other neurological sign of distress, as I'd feared. All eyes looked to me for instruction as the head man said, "We don't really know whether to take him to emergency, or what."

"Let's go ahead and get him in the ambulance, and see what they say at the hospital," I said, surprising myself at the calmness of my demeanor, my racing heart slowing with the evidence that my father was still alive.

As I supported my father down the hallway, with an attendant on the other side, my dad began to sob.

"What's wrong Daddy?" I asked.

"I—I won't ever be coming back here," he said, then started to tremble. "I'll n-never see my home again." Tears began streaming down his cheeks, and his body seemed to sag as he gave utterance to his greatest fear.

I nearly broke down myself, hearing this semblance of lucidity and understanding come from someplace within my father's dementia, his tears streaming as he seemed to sag in our arms after giving utterance to a possibility that surely terrified him. The probability that he might well be right tore through to my core, as well.

"No, Daddy, that's not true. We're taking you to the hospital just for some tests, and you'll be back here tomorrow," I said to comfort him, though I knew it might not be true. As I helped put my father into the ambulance, his sobbing words began a reverberation in my mind that would continue to haunt me during the coming days.

I won't ever see my home again.

Pop's words were still in my mind as I sat in vigil beside his hospital bed, after the four hours in the emergency room and conversations with doctors who told me they had found no signs of a stroke, that hopefully Pop was only reacting to a urinary tract infection. *"I—I'll never see my home again, I'll never see my home again."*

The words haunted me during the five days of his hospitalization. Pop failed to respond to medication, and a couple of times I had to help nurses restrain his arms as he tried to pull out his IV lines. He often repeated, "I've got to go home to see about Marguerite," or "I've got to go home to see about my wife." I was moved to tears that this man's first duty, even in the depths of dementia, would still be predicated on the love for his wife.

The sorrowful scene was embellished tenfold in my writer's imagination, replaying over and over in my head while I wiped sweat from his fevered brow and the spittle from his mouth as he ranted. He believed he was in a funeral home somewhere up on Route 58, ominously confusing the hospital with the nursing home where his sister Sarah had once been and saying repeatedly that soon his son would be there to take him home, oblivious to the fact that I was there beside him.

His words were still torturing me—*I will never see my home again*—as I told the social worker, in the doorway to my father's room, that she should proceed with preparing the papers for his commitment to a nursing home. In the background Pop, now tied to his bed to restrain him from pulling out the IVs, exclaimed, "I—I'm not worried about being at this funeral home, 'cause Derrell brought me here, and I *know* he's coming to pick me up."

It seemed as if my worst fears were coming to pass when the social worker told me that the only nursing home with a bed available was the god-awful place his Aunt Sarah had been just before she had died, only two months before.

I felt an ebb and flow from terror to numbness during the hours spent beside Pop's bed. On one hand, I had to continue to love the human being lost in delirium who remained my father, while trying to make sure disinterested nurses took proper care of him, as I took care of the little/not-so-little things like putting salve on legs scaled by eczema and washing and treating feet darkened and, to my horror, smelling from an absence of attention given to his condition by his caregivers—doctors, nurses, and home caregivers. Even I felt guilt in not having known about it, not paying enough attention.

At the same time, I had to work at being objective, pragmatic: *Your father is in no shape to return home, so get ready to do what you have to do.*

But a deep dread of the nursing home decision was all-consuming, most especially with my father's frightened words and the image of his tears still filling my brain. *Stay calm,* I would tell myself, when Pop would awaken to see my face there beside him with a look of recognition and love—such love as I'd never seen from him—the love now like that of a child for his parent, a love that embodied hope amid delirium when he looked up and asked me, "When are we going home, Derrell? I'm tired of being in this funeral home."

During my bedside vigils, I would flash back to those prison days, could not help but think of Pop's long drives with Mama to distant prisons, to see me every month. I remembered those moments when there was not much to talk about, when the three of us would simply sit in silence. Moments when I received comfort from just their *presence* and from memories of the devotion they gave to me, their wayward child, for so many years.

Though I'd known it all along, I now *felt* it: it was their love and devotion that had sustained me during those twenty years inside. It was their uncommon loyalty that had given me a chance at redemption. And while I might have felt a modicum of satisfaction at being there for them, as they'd been for me, I now had to make a decision that filled me with an unimaginable dread: I had to commit my father to an *institution,* commit him to a nursing home, a place that, in my mind, was actually a *prison*—a prison where he would surely die.

And so it was that I instructed Karen the social worker, a sweet, African-American woman with freckles: *Go ahead and prepare the papers.* She then had to locate a home for placement, as the hospital covered only care needed immediately and then they more or less forced a discharge upon you. Pop had gone in on a Sunday night, and the doctor scheduled his release for a Friday. On Thursday morning I called Uncle Julian, who by now had become the legal guardian for my parents, and told him to be prepared to come in on Friday to sign Pop out and then to travel with us to the nursing home.

Then on Friday, when Pop was awakened for lunch, he looked over at me, then looked around, and with a degree of cogency asked, "How long have I been in the hospital?"

I could not believe it. "Do you know where you are, Daddy?"

"Yes," he said, "this is Memorial Hospital, ain't it?" I told him that indeed it was and asked if he knew where the hospital was located. "Why you ask me that? Of course, I know. We're just up the street from your house."

It was miraculous. He sat up and ate every bit of his lunch, lucidly asking me how Mama was, and if I was going to take him home later that day. I told him that the doctors wanted to keep him one more day, and that then he would be able to go home.

I stayed with him all of the day and into the evening, to make sure this seeming recovery wasn't a fluke. I arrived at the hospital early the next morning and found that he was in some semblance of his right mind, still knew where he was, and was still anxious to go home to see about Mama.

My father's doctor told me that evidently he had just been thrown out of kilter from having had a urinary tract infection. "When a patient has Alzheimer's, anything that goes wrong with the body can throw them into delirium," he said.

When I talked to the social worker, she suggested that I go ahead with commitment. "He's going to have to go sooner or later," she said, "and, while I hate to say it, sooner is usually better—not only for him, so he can get adjusted while he still has some of his faculties. But moreover, I'm thinking about you. I see what you've been going through, and I've seen hundreds of situations with caregivers, with all of the stress. And I hate to tell you, many of them end up passing away *before* the ones they're giving care to. You need to think about looking out for yourself, too."

We were in a tiny, closed meeting room, just off the corridor, near the nurses' station for the floor. It was smaller than some of the prison cells I'd seen, and I felt closed in.

"I need to make a call and talk with my uncle. He is the legal guardian and conservator, and he'll have to come in to sign the papers," I told the young woman. But I really needed to just get out of the room. I asked her if she could wait there a moment while I stepped out to make the call.

Walking down to the end of the hallway, where there was a bit of light coming in from a window, I noted that all the halls were painted in shades I knew very well, various gradations of what I call "institutional pastels"—bland greens and blues, or beige. I realized that the same sanitized colors, scientifically processed to reduce madness on submarines, would be what Pop would be seeing in a nursing facility. The landscape man would never again see the lush greens of the land that had been passed down from his father's farm, where he'd built his home.

By the time I reached the window, I had made my decision. I pulled the cell phone from my pocket, called Uncle Julian, and told him he needn't come. I was taking Pop home.

* * *

Several months later, Mama was hospitalized with what appeared to be a stroke. After a week of hospitalization and a desperate search for

35

a bed in a nursing home, I called the prosecutor who had called for the max in my case—life, for the armed robbery I had committed—but was also instrumental in my making parole. We had become friends, in a sense, after my release. He made a call to one of the best nursing facilities in the city, where his mother had been, and I was able to get Mama into a place called Roman Eagle. It was an irony that, by befriending a one-time antagonist, I found that he would bring his influence to bear and come to our rescue.

Still, taking Mama out of the hospital and committing her to the nursing home filled me with sorrow and guilt. For a while I felt compelled to visit her every day and found that doing things for her like helping her to eat, or doing her nails, brought out a certain tenderness in me. But I soon realized that I couldn't continue to go see her every day.

Though she had begun to do much better than had been the case when she was at home, I was still wracked with guilt every day that I did not visit. I tried to make up for missed days by paying a private sitter to keep her company, but this began exhausting the available funds, because Pop's round-the-clock care had continued. Though heartened by improvement, visits to see her left me even more depressed. The pain of seeing her struggle to walk again—with the belief that walking would enable her to return to her home—was heartrending every time I was there.

I sank deeper into depression, as I felt as if I had failed, in not making enough money with my writing, to keep her at home. And the feeling of failure mounted as the family spent the remaining funds we had available to take care of Pop—confronting me with the necessity of placing him in the nursing home with Mama, not because he was "so bad off" that he needed to be there but because there was no longer enough money to keep someone round the clock in the home. I had cousins who thought that I should move in with him and take care of him, but I knew that was not an option for my sanity, much less my life as a writer.

I felt helpless in the face of my next great decision: I would have to, in effect, have my father locked away in an institution. And again,

I could not help but feel that I would be putting my father into a prison.

* * *

I have to put my father in the nursing home was the guilt-inducing, constant thought in my life. I felt like the decision was killing me.

For some reason I recalled images of my father from my childhood: driving his tractor on hills on the land where I grew up, sometimes actually plowing fields and grading land *standing up.* Other scenes of him from my childhood in the country came to mind: my father with his father's single-barreled shotgun, teaching me to hunt; working with him gathering bales of straw in the fields; learning to drive *on* his tractor, at age ten; working in winters with him cutting pulp wood trees, then trucking them to the saw mill on the other side of the town.

And I had my memories from just seven years before, when I got out: he was still in fine physical shape, still running his landscaping company, still a handsome seventy-six. He was still doing what amounted to landscape architecture, sculpting the land with his tractors, vigorous and exacting. And, Deacon Hopkins would still stand tall in church, leading the congregation in prayer—a fine figure of a man.

We bonded more than ever before, during that time, often travelling the eighty miles from Danville to Duke University, where I had doctors do his initial diagnosis and treatment for the Alzheimer's. And for a while we worked together, when I took over a big job landscaping a bank, with him marveling, proudly, at how I was able to read and execute the landscape architect's plans.

All that seemed to remain of my father now was a shell, the brain matter, the cortex filled with protein tangles and tau malformation, the imprint of Alzheimer's, allowing him to live on as Daniel Hopkins but little more. Memories of my son Roderick exist there, in his mind, and in mine—along with the pain of Rod's sudden passing, from a heart condition, when he was but twelve—some fifteen years before.

I began to think of Rod a lot during this time, because he had looked somewhat like my father, and I have kept a treasured Polaroid of the three of us (taken in front of a prison visiting room vending machine) on my writing desk. Nowadays, it seemed like every look from my father, as I withdrew from his presence, reminded me of the longing I remembered in Rod's eyes when I left him with his mother or saw him leave after visits in various prisons. I sensed the same with my father giving me the same long looks when I'd leave after visiting him out in the country.

It seemed as if I could always sense a bit of anger and bewilderment at my leaving, my leaving equating to treachery, all that was now happening around him coming down to a sense of blame upon me, that it was *my* fault. At the same time, there was an unqualified love I could feel when he saw me.

I realized, in one of those moments that, ironically, I had now become *his* father figure. This realization, mixed with both guilt and moral obligation, gave me a new sense of purpose, and became a balm of sorts, for the loneliness of my existence in Danville.

* * *

The tune on the radio was Miles Davis's "All Blues," next switching up to "Blue in Green." I was blue, and in deep, psychic pain. I could not help but wonder, *I endured so much, why must I go through still more, alone?*

It was time to get out of the house, to go for a long walk, hope that the air of spring might rejuvenate me. I headed east, stopping by my analyst's office for an unscheduled visit, thinking that one of the few niceties of living in a small city is that you might actually have your analyst's office but a block around the corner.

Back before things had gotten worse for him, I had taken Pop to see a neuro-psychologist, because of his complaints of "dizziness." After a series of visits and tests, she told me, "There's not much I can do to help your father. It's just the progression of the disease. But I've noticed you seem a little stressed out. Maybe you'd like to come in for some therapy?"

Telling her now during this impromptu visit about the struggle I was having concerning my father, she offered her opinion: "He will probably be disoriented when you put him in the nursing home and go downhill." *Thanks a f**kin' lot*, I think. Then she added, "It will probably be better that he go in while his wife is still there." Thanks again, for raising the idea that Mama is not guaranteed to be around much longer. "That is, *if* you are lucky enough to place him there." Now I *really* appreciated that one. Food for thought—or worry, depending on one's mindset.

Walking back up West Main, my mind searching for an anchor, I thought that maybe I needed to take heart in the struggle of it all, to look upon the situation as if I were still a member of the Black Panther Party, working to free myself of the fetters of everyday life, so that my work might someday soar into the consciousness of humanity (or less grandly, maybe make a bit of difference in the world).

As I passed the Averett University Library the scent of the magnolias there held me for a moment, and I decided to go inside. Students were at work on computers. As I walked among the shelves I thought of the three college readers in which my work had already been published, and visualized students in libraries all over the country being able to pull the book I was writing from the shelves, or studying my words in class. I thought of how some lost and searching young prisoner might one day encounter my book on the shelf and obtain some hope.

When I was fighting against the idea of closing down the landscaping business my father had founded, my analyst had told me, "You have to realize that people might soon forget your father's business, but they will remember him for many years if you get your book in print."

Maybe this is how my father—my family, my son—will have to live on? I thought. *Yeah, I like that thought. I have to break free; I cannot worry myself to death about my father. He will have to live on through me, just as my son has had to*—which made me flash back on the dream in which my son's spirit had merged into my body.

The weight of those thoughts converted to still more pressure upon me to concentrate upon my writing in the future, but at that moment, I wanted to get away from such thinking, get outside once more, onto the sidewalks of Danville.

As I walked, the refrain from a Curtis Mayfield song filled my brain: "*Got to keep on pushin'. . . Long as I have the strength . . .*" The tune brought to mind the one Alzheimer's support group meeting I'd gone to some months before. It had been too much for me, all the shit those people were going through I did not want to imagine, couldn't bear to imagine.

But the words of this one black lady who was there remained embedded in my memory. After describing the wandering, rambling, damn-near oblivious behavior of her husband, she had said, "I took care of him for nearly ten years, now. And if God gives me the strength, I'll take care of him for ten more." So what was my duty now—should I have less determination for my father?

I wondered that maybe my openness to feeling had made me soft since my release from prison, that maybe I needed some of that hard-ass gangster revolutionary shit running through my veins again. *You've been livin' like your heart is pumpin' Kool-Aid or somethin'*, I told myself. *Maybe it's time for you to get hard again.*

On the walk back home I encountered David, an old associate from my days "in the street," who, with age, had straightened up, and begun a walking program. (As fate would have it, this was the brother who had sold me the bullets for my Magnum the night of the foolish heist that had netted me the life sentence.)

Retired from the street life now, he asked about my father, whom he knew from growing up in the black community called Brucetown with us. I told him of the dilemma I was facing with Pop perhaps having to go into the nursing home with Mom. "I'm not tryin' to tell you what to do," he said to me, "but usually when they go into the nursing home, they don't come out. It's all downhill from there."

Now I *really* didn't want to hear this, so I quickly broke off the conversation, and as I made my way home, I remembered how Mama had told me, during my last year at Nottoway Prison, "I just want to stay alive until you make it back home." I had helped to extend her life, and Pop's, for the five years I'd been back; and though friends and family members would say to me nice things like, "God bless you, Derrell, for all you're doing for your folks," I still felt as if I hadn't done enough. And now, thinking of what David had just said to me, I wondered if, after all this, I was now about to put my father into a nursing home, to die.

*　*　*

I sank, once more, into a depression as deep as any I'd experienced, and began to worry about my own psychological survival. I was unable to write, unable to relive the pain of my past while beset with such guilt as I was feeling. Filled with anxiety, I found that I was afraid to *feel anything,* blaming myself for being weak, having become soft from having opened myself up to emotion in the wider world in which I lived, wondering how I might call upon the Panther resolve of my youth—or even some of the gangster coldness—that might alleviate the psychological pain I was experiencing. I would watch movies on television and would break down into tears whenever one struck a sensitive chord, as when one film about a man who had lost his family in an accident, while driving, visited their graves at the end of the movie. I tried then to write about my own visit to the cemetery where my son was buried and struggled to fight through the continuing grief, but was so overcome I could only lie down in a fetal position, praying for the relief of sleep.

And indeed, as it had been while I was in prison, sleep became my refuge—the only freedom I seemed to know, to paraphrase the pop song "Wildflower." I spent days just struggling to get out of bed, and rarely left the house. The isolation I was experiencing with the book was sometimes worse than what I'd had to deal with in prison. At least there I'd had to go to the chow hall at least once a day and encounter people. During this period, while struggling to write, I would spend days without talking to *anyone* and even began calling for delivery of Chinese food, just so I wouldn't have to go out.

The situation became so bad that I knew I had to do something. A visit one evening by an old acquaintance from my days of reefer madness served as a wake-up call. After I let him into my living room, he opened up his palm to show me two rocks of crack cocaine. "You can do one of them, if you don't mind me doing the other," he said, bringing out a pipe from his pocket.

For the briefest moment, I considered taking the road to darkness I'd avoided since my return; and in that moment, I realized that I was in danger, in danger for having weakened in my resolve for even five seconds. I opened the door for the man who had once been a friend and said, "I think you better leave, Bruh. And maybe try to get some help. But don't come here anymore, unless you're straight."

I recalled the pledge I'd taken in jail, not only to stay away from illegal drugs but to never take prescription antidepressants. But that was before the age of drugs like Prozac, and having read about the positive effects such medication was having upon millions, I decided to consult my doctor and give it a try.

My doctor told me, "You're obviously depressed, and have been for some time. Try these samples and let me know if it helps. You'll feel icky for a week or two, but then the drug should begin to help you." My physician was British and sometimes used what was rather quaint terminology to describe possible side effects

After one week of side effects, I still felt messed up. I had to call Shelia—the girlfriend in Richmond who would one day become my wife—and cancel my weekend visit. I tried to explain that I'd decided to try medication for my depression, something she did not want to understand, for she thought that she—and our love—should be able to get me through anything. (People who have not suffered clinical depression can never seem to understand it as being a physical condition of the brain rather than something you should just be able to "get over" in time.)

After weeks of taking the medication, however, I still didn't feel any better and was perhaps even more depressed because I was *still* depressed. And being forced to make my decision about Pop did not help. The day when I finally made myself take him for his preliminary physical to the physician who would admit him to Roman Eagle seemed to sap all energy from my body, left me with the feeling that I was unable to breathe in the humid summer air as we left the doctor's office. I now had my father on the waiting list for the nursing home, and it almost seemed as if I were waiting for the internment of my own soul.

I would take him to spend hours with Mama in the hope that he would get used to being at the nursing home and be better able to adjust, once he was admitted. But he wasn't having any of it. When I broached the idea of his going there to be with Mama, he'd rail. "I've got a home that I had built from the ground up, and paid for," he would say. "And I'm in good shape—I'm not nursing home material."

I had to dismiss all of the caregivers except Anita, who began staying with Pop around the clock. Then, seeing what I was going through, Anita told me one day, "You can let your father come stay with me, in my home. I'll take care of him, and he won't have to go into Roman Eagle."

I was relieved. Anita's house was even nicer than my folk's home in the country, and it then became a matter of getting Pop to go along with the transition, which was not an easy thing. "We'll have to take him there, to spend a few nights," I told her, "and then just let him know that he won't be going back home."

And so it happened that my father, Daniel Hopkins, came to reside in the modest home of Mrs. Anita Tomasso, a New Jersey widow whose roots were in Danville, who cared for him with love for the next six years. During this time, I was able to finish and publish my memoir, marry Shelia, and move to Richmond, returning periodically to see him. "I don't have no aches, nor pain," he told me one day, in his mid-eighties. The hard physical work of landscaping had kept his body and heart strong. Shortly after we moved him I came across a new drug, from Germany—Memantine—that worked small wonders for him for a few years. (The neurologist marveled: "It's like he's better than he was two years ago.") So Daddy still remembered my name, recognized my face during visits, and he kept his weight up with the good cooking for which Anita prided herself. Remarkably, however, the deacon lost all of the dogma of religion but grew more philosophical.

I took him to visit the grave of his mother, once, out in the country where a church cemetery dating back to slavery had been uncovered and preserved. During the car trip back to Anita's, out of the blue, while looking ahead into the distance, came this: "You know, Derrell, we don't do this for them. We do this for ourselves." What do you mean? I asked. "They are gone, they don't know we were there, that we came to see their graves. So we do this for ourselves," he repeated. "To make US feel good—like we have done something for somebody else."

This philosophical outlook lasted to his dying day, it would seem. "The night that he passed,' Anita would tell me, "I went by his room to check on him and say goodnight again. I said, 'Guess what, Mr. Hopkins? Michael Jackson died last night.' He looked up at me, standing in the doorway, and I could tell he knew who Michael Jackson was. And you know what he said? He said, 'We all have to go, sometimes, and he laid his head back down.'" And so it was that my father passed peacefully in his sleep, as they say, on June 26, 2009. . . . In his own room. In his own bed.

BUTTER IN THE SUGAR BOWL

An Excerpt from *Not for Everyday Use*

ELIZABETH NUNEZ

When did my father begin his gradual decline? He had retired early from the Shell Oil Company, when he was only fifty-seven. Our island Trinidad had gained its independence from Britain, and the oilmen from England, Holland, and America who owned the company had begun divesting their holdings, aware that it would only be a matter of time before the island would take control of its natural resources. They gave my father a generous severance package, but he continued to work as a labor consultant for decades afterward, representing private and public interests in the Industrial Court in Trinidad and at the International Labour Organization in Geneva, where he was already well known during his years working for both the colonial government and Shell.

Then one day he was putting butter in his tea. I was there to see him do it.

We were having breakfast, and I asked him if he wanted more sugar. "I'll get it," he said, and stuck his spoon in the butter dish.

I reached to help him, but my mother stopped me. "He just wants your attention," she said angrily. "He knows perfectly well what he is doing."

Did he?

Ten years ago, I made the trip to Columbus, Mississippi, to see my parents. They were visiting my brother Gregory and his wife Beverly. My mother had passed the five-year threshold for breast cancer survivors, and she wanted to travel again. She chose to visit Gregory, I think not only because he is a doctor and she felt more comfortable being in his home in case her illness flared up again, but also because she had a soft spot for this son of hers who had endured the blows she had rained on his bottom and legs. No longer in constant fear that my father's paltry salary from the colonial government, together with the little money she managed to eke out from her domestic poultry farm, would not be enough to feed her ever-expanding brood, my mother became more relaxed as she grew older. At the same time, however, she was tortured by guilt that she had been too hard on us, especially on Gregory. I think especially Gregory, because, unlike the rest of us, he never got angry with her; he never pouted; he never gave her the silent treatment for days, which was my specialty.

Gregory took his blows without rancor, but he continued to play tricks on my mother. After a ruse where he called the house pretending to be promoting a new refrigerator, there were others. My mother was always fooled. She never seemed able to detect Gregory's voice under the foreign accents he used, but in her defense I would say that my brother was a master of vocal disguise. He also made her laugh, particularly when she got frustrated with the mistakes she constantly made trying to sew dresses for my sisters and me. Somehow, she rarely seemed able to fit sleeves in the armholes she had cut out from the fabric; either she made them too big or too small. Gregory would help her out of her predicament. "Rip them out, Mum, rip them out," he would say, joining forces with her. "Your machine telling you it too hot for sleeves." My mother would burst out laughing, and together they would start pulling seams apart. Pieces of cloth would go flying into the air.

My parents seemed happy when I saw them in the bucolic setting of Gregory's home in Mississippi. The tall leafy trees, the green grass, the gently undulating hills, the intermittent whistle of birds as they glided through the warm, turgid air must have reminded them of tropical Trinidad. The first morning I was there my father wanted me to go walking with him, to show me the birds he had identified in the woods. Trailing behind my father on the road that sloped gently down from my brother's home and then steeply up before descending again, I was huffing and puffing with every ascent. Even at eighty-three my father was a brisk walker. He could climb to the top of a hill without pausing for breath.

The year before, my father had driven me up the winding road to the Asa Wright bird sanctuary in the dense rainforest of the northern mountain range in Trinidad. The area, once known as the Spring Hill Estate, used to be a thriving cocoa plantation, but the cocoa industry had dried up when oil was discovered in the south of the island. Asa and Newcombe Wright, the owners of Spring Hill, turned the estate into a sanctuary for wildlife. It became particularly well known for the rare birds that nested in the forest trees. At one point 159 species of birds were recorded there. My father loved going to Asa Wright. The day I went with him he shamed me and a group of bird lovers, some half his age, by trotting up the inclines while most of us had to take breaks to catch our breath. I discovered my father had gone to the bird sanctuary so many times the workers there knew him well enough to address him by name. We had lunch in the dining room, and the cook came out of the kitchen to greet him. "Red beans and rice again, Mr. Nunez?" the man asked. As far as I could see, there were no red beans and rice on the cafeteria-style counter, but stewed red beans and rice are what my father had for lunch.

My father loved birds, his interest ignited by his forest warden father who was himself influenced by his Portuguese father who had chosen to work on the cocoa plantation rather than follow his Portuguese compatriots into the dry-goods business. So intimate was my father's relationship with the birds in Trinidad, he could call out to them in their distinctive whistles and they would respond in kind. In the early days, my father used this skill to trap the birds. He would whistle to them, luring them to the branch of a tree he had lined with *laglee*, a gluey substance. When the birds alighted on the branch, they would get stuck and my father would pluck them out and cage them. I had grown up with birdcages dangling from wires attached to the ceiling of our porch. Then, surprisingly, when I returned home from college, the cages were no longer there. My father had set the birds free. He did the same with his fish, though the empty tank still remained where it was, a reminder I presume he wanted of the thoughtlessness of his youth. The disappearance of those cages and that empty fish tank would be a lesson to me. Though my father did not give me an explanation for what he had done, his unspoken message was clear: we had no right to take a living creature out of its natural habitat just to serve our pleasure.

In those days, as now, my father's joy came from looking and "talking" to the birds, he in his habitat, they in theirs. All along that country road in Columbus, Mississippi, my father whistled to the American birds, as he had done with the birds in Trinidad, and they whistled back to him. My father seemed vigorous and alert, in full control of his enormous intellect. I was certain my mother was right. The butter in the tea was my father's call for attention. Nothing was wrong with his brain.

Confident that he had been simply toying with me, I decided to seek his help with a problem that had been troubling me. Gregory was a chain-smoker. Nothing I said or did seemed to convince him that he should stop smoking, not my alarm at his constant dry cough nor the statistics I recited to him on lung cancer and heart disease.

"Gregory's house is practically blue with smoke," I complained to my father.

I had said the same to my brother, and he countered, "When we were children, our house was always blue with smoke and we survived."

It was true. We had survived, and all of us apparently in good health. My father was a chain-smoker too. For sixteen years growing up in my parents' home, I rarely saw my father without a cigarette. We lived in the tropics, so our windows were always open, yet our house was suffused with the stink of cigarettes; it was embedded in the furniture and in our clothes. Cigarette ashes were piled up everywhere in saucers and ashtrays. I still remember the colorful plastic ashtrays I bought for my father for Christmas and his birthday. They were the best gifts I could think of giving him.

"Dad is eighty-three," Gregory reminded me. "Statistics don't tell the truth for everyone."

But our father did not wake up every morning with a racking cough.

Now, as we climbed the incline toward Gregory's house, I pleaded with my father to speak to him. My father slowed down and faced me. "I am to blame," he said softly. "I set a bad example."

I tried to convince him he was wrong. "But you stopped. Gregory could have learned that from you too."

"Gregory was already a man when I stopped," he replied.

This was not accurate. Gregory was not yet a man when my father stopped smoking. He was fourteen, still a child, when he first began pilfering my father's cigarettes. The ones he stole from my father were not the filtered type; those had not yet reached our island. There was no wad at the bottom to dilute some of the poisons that would course through the smoker's lungs. The cigarettes my father inhaled, sucking the dark smoke deep into his lungs, were unfiltered. I know because I bought cartons of unfiltered cigarettes for him in the duty-free shops every time I returned to Trinidad on holiday.

My father stopped smoking in his mid-fifties, abruptly and without forethought, though he would say that he had tried to stop years before then. He was on the sea this time, in an open pirogue with his godson, a young man in his early teens. They were out fishing. The sun was beating down on their heads, and my father, perhaps to ease the sting of the sun burning his flesh, sought comfort in the familiar pleasure of smoking. He dug into his pocket, took out a cigarette, and lit it. According to his version of the story, his godson turned to him and made this innocent request: "Uncle, why you don't throw that cigarette in the sea?" And that is exactly what my father did. He threw the lit cigarette into the sea and never touched another one again.

"It is the one major regret in my life," my father said to me as I quickened my pace to catch up with him. "I taught my sons to smoke."

I reminded him that his sons were men now. If Gregory wanted, he could get help to break the habit.

My father shook his head sadly. "I would be the happiest person in the world if Gregory would quit. He is such a good son to me."

I did not see then that my father's eyes had become misty, or notice, as we approached the house, that the jauntiness had gone out of his stride. I was too distracted by the presence of my brother's car in the driveway, thrilled that he had come home for lunch. If my father had set a bad example for his sons with his cigarette habit, he had set a good one as a man who put his family before his ambitions, for I had no doubt that Gregory had to reschedule his patients' appointments to be here with us in time for lunch.

My father did not have patients, of course, but he was an ambitious young man, a junior officer at the Ministry of Labour, with his eye on the top of the ladder, a not-unfounded possibility for a non-European in the days just before independence, and yet he risked that ambition to have lunch with his children almost every day when we were in school.

My father eventually made it to the top of the ladder. He was in his early forties when he was appointed commissioner of labor. The previous commissioner, Solomon Hochoy, was the first nonwhite British governor of Trinidad and Tobago. Later, when our island gained independence, he was made governor general and knighted by the Queen of England. Though Sir Solomon had not achieved this status when my father worked in the ministry, the signs were already there that he was favored by the British. It was also likely that if any local man was to rise in the British colonial government, it would be someone attached to the Ministry of Labour, which was the first of the ministries the British colonial government had more or less entrusted to locals. Two world wars, the failing sugarcane economy, and the persistent drumbeat for decolonization across the globe had made the British skittish. If problems came, they would come from the labor force. Better to have one of the people's own in charge of the labor ministry when the onslaught rumbled through the island.

So it was not at all far-fetched for us to assume that our father's future looked very bright indeed. Yet every day my father left his office at lunchtime to pick us up from school. I was at Tranquility Girls School then, the equivalent of American middle school. Yolande and Richard were in high school, she at the prestigious St. Joseph's

Convent for girls, and he on scholarship at the equally prestigious St. Mary's College for boys. David and Jacqueline were in elementary school. At around noon, soon after my school broke for lunch, I would see my father turning the corner in his sky-blue Rambler, one of the perks of his position as commissioner of labor. He would already have picked up Yolande and Richard, and after getting me, he would go for David and Jacqueline. How he managed to do this, I have no idea. I cannot imagine that all his affairs at the ministry ended just before noon, or that a meeting with a superior would be conveniently scheduled to allow him to go home at exactly that time. It must have been risky for him to leave his office, and yet he rarely failed. Sometimes he was late, but always I knew the Rambler would be turning the corner and soon I would be having lunch with him, my mother, and my siblings.

Family comes first, my father said. And so Gregory was following in his father's footsteps. He would drop everything, reschedule his patients' appointments, and have lunch with his mother and father.

The house was thrumming with happy voices when we came into the dining room. My sister-in-law, Beverly, who is Jamaican, had made *pelau* for lunch. *Pelau* is a quintessential Trinidadian dish which locals contend only they know how to make properly. My mother had apparently just complimented Beverly on the tenderness of the chicken and the graininess of the rice, and Gregory, who was sitting at the head of the table, was grinning from ear to ear with pride. Next to his hand was a lit cigarette resting on an ashtray, already burned halfway down and sending a thin trail of smoke across the table. As he got up to greet our father, Gregory reached for the cigarette and was about to put it to his lips when I pounced on him. "Do you know how miserable you are making Daddy?" I yelled. "He said the greatest regret in his life is that you are still smoking. My God, don't you care about him?" More accusations flew out of my mouth like venom.

My father sat down heavily in his chair. "I am to blame," he murmured. And for the first time I noticed the moisture in his eyes.

Gregory put down his cigarette, threw me a scathing look, and then turned his back on me. "So, Dad," he began as if I had not said a word to him, "how was your day? Catch any birds? Picoplat? Chikechong?" He smiled at my father adoringly.

In an instant, my father's mood changed. "I saw one today," he chirped. His face brightened.

"A picoplat?"

"No, a semp. A really nice one. Bright yellow feathers on his breast. Black streaks too."

"And the wings?"

"White. The brightest white you ever saw."

"Did you whistle to him?"

"Yes. And he whistled back."

I simmered with indignation. There were no picoplats, chikechongs, or semps in Mississippi. Those were tropical birds. But I stifled my anger. My father looked too happy, and I was loath to extinguish the light shining with increasing brightness in his eyes.

Back and forth my brother and father went talking about semps, picoplats, and chikechongs, about which had the brightest feathers, which made the sweetest music. Then suddenly my father turned to me. "You saw the semp too, didn't you, Elizabeth?"

What could I say? Could I deny him the joy of remembering his days in the forest singing with the birds? Before I could think up an answer, he began to whistle, an exact imitation of the song of the yellow-feathered semp. I didn't know what to do, what to say. I gestured to my brother for help. He whistled back as if he were a semp too, and for a while he and my father continued this way, with call and response, until abruptly my father stopped waiting for my brother's response. Now his whistles became shriller, louder, more frantic.

"Dad." My brother moved closer to him. I could tell he was getting nervous. "Dad."

My father continued to whistle.

"Dad!"

My father pursed his lips to whistle again, but this time no sound came out of his mouth. "It's my fault," he murmured. He hung down his head. "I'm to blame. My fault."

My mother placed her hand on his arm. "Come, Waldo." She tugged his arm gently.

My father glanced over at her.

"Waldo," my mother crooned. "Come now. Let's go. It's time for a nap."

So she knew. So my mother was aware that my father was drifting away. Her anger with me when I tried to still his hand as he reached for the butter to put in his tea was really her terror, her fear that she could be losing her partner in life, the man who had traveled with her through all the sorrows, joys, failures, and triumphs of their more than sixty years together. She had said my father made a conscious decision to give up. He would not allow himself to be taken by surprise; he would be ready when the Grim Reaper came. My father was pretending to be weak, she said, shuffling back and forth through the house like a senile old man, but I know now she was the one pretending, hoping against hope she was right.

ANCHORED AGAINST ALZHEIMER'S
SONSYREA TATE

The evening Grandma punched Granddad in the face so hard he stumbled was a pivotal moment for me. Instinctively, he tried to strike back. "Stop it! Both of you! Stop it!" I yelled, wedged between them as they clawed at each other's clothes and faces. I clutched Grandma's wrists in my hands the way my mother had recently taught me, but she kicked at Granddad with all she had. "Stop it!" I repeated. I felt like a six-year-old child—but I had to be stronger and wiser for all of us at this moment. I pushed Granddad back, and Grandma punched him again.

I stayed between them.

"Granddad, give me your necktie!" I demanded. I managed to get Granddad's necktie off his neck and wrap it around Grandma's wrists. I pulled her into the living room and forced her onto the couch, and noticed Granddad doubled-over trying to catch his breath. Grandma fought to get free from me; I sat on her. Fearing me in a way she had never feared me before, Grandma tried to spit on me in self-defense. "Jesus!" she yelled. I untied her wrists, and I jumped up off her as she called out to her savior, a savior she'd been taught to love and trust in her youth, a savior she had worshipped in song, speech, and life choices ever since I could remember.

"Jesus!" Grandma, ninety-five, cried like a baby, yelling, sobbing, shoulders slumped. "Jesus! You said you'd never forsake me! Why have you forsaken me?" she cried.

Granddad stood in the wide-open doorway, dazed, tears streaming down his face. He had promised Grandma, who had Alzheimer's, he would never put her in a nursing home. I had heard them make that promise to each other when I was in my twenties. Now in my forties, I would do all I could to help keep them together in their own home. Sometimes it was hard.

"Jesus! Come and take me! Loooooooord, come and get me!" Grandma pleaded.

We were in the midst of a "sun-downing" moment, the time of day around sunset when an individual with Alzheimer's gets particularly agitated and disoriented. I had learned about managing sunset moments a year earlier but had not yet mastered the process of dealing with it. On this day, I had taken my grandparents to my baby brother's wedding. They were happy to go, and I figured their very presence, as an elderly couple, would inspire and encourage others. In quiet conversations before and after the wedding, I would enjoy reminding family and friends that they had eloped right after high school graduation and remained married seventy-five years later.

Privately, however, the storm of Grandma's Alzheimer's disease had shredded my idyllic perception of their love and my perception of them. I had idolized my grandparents, but this silent apocalypse had laid them bare. Turns out they were as imperfect as me. I couldn't tell anyone, of course, the secrets this disease was exposing. On Facebook I simply posted, "Love is beautiful—except when it ain't."

Grandma and Granddad had enjoyed my brother's picture-perfect outdoor wedding, held on a scenic hilltop beneath clear blue skies and sunshine. They had smiled and been hugged all afternoon. I had pulled them away to leave before the celebration was over to avoid exhausting them, but when I got them home, it was clear that I had kept them out too long. Granddad and I struggled getting Grandma out of the car and into the house, and as soon as we closed the door behind us in the house, Grandma's tirade began as she insisted on leaving the house. Initially, she had hollered for the police. "Poleeeeeeece! Heeeeeelp! They're trying to kill me. Heeeeeeelp!" But in the final phase of her fit, she called out to her beloved Christ. Her call to Christ awakened my inner spirit, and I went to war.

"OUR Father, who art in heaven! HALLOWED be thy name!

THY Kingdom come! THY will be done! On earth, as it is in heaven." I began shouting the Lord's Prayer on repeat, pacing in a circle through the house because this had worked for the past few years. Sometimes Grandma would settle down as soon as she recognized the familiar words. Other times I would pray and pace for close to an hour to calm her. The prayer also settled Granddad and gave me peace. Depending on the severity and time of Grandma's storm, I would recite the prayer in steady moderate tones or yell it at the top of my lungs.

It never failed to calm Grandma—and anchor me too. When the Alzheimer's-induced storms of wild violence or quiet disorientation raged, threatening to flatten anybody in their path, the familiar and reverent sound of the Lord's Prayer saved the day.

But sometimes I feared I was losing my own mind. I was afraid I was looking and sounding like a religious fanatic. Even Granddad, a devout Christian and deacon in his church, seemed puzzled and worried at the sight and sound of my fervent prayer. I had never seen him go into war-like prayer. I had never seen anyone in my family, which is very religious, do this. Our religion had been Sunday service for the Christians, daily salats for the Muslims, and other rituals on occasion. But Grandma's Alzheimer's served as a storm that ripped away the pretense of religion for me. I was learning that prayer is more than a neat, tidy little tradition. Prayer is power. In the middle of the night when neither Granddad nor the overnight aide could manage Grandma, my recitation of the Lord's Prayer prevailed.

On that fateful night after the wedding when Grandma's whirlwind hit with more force than usual, the Lord's Prayer won. Grandma eventually whimpered out.

"Come on, baby. Let's get you to bed. You know I love you," Granddad said tenderly, taking Grandma by the hand and leading her upstairs. I plopped down on a chair in the dining room and turned on the Gospel Music Channel to continue filling the house with the familiar sounds of unquestioning faith. Douglas Miller's song, "My Soul Has Been Anchored in the Lord," came on, and I almost broke down in tears. Now I knew what this song meant. Grandma's soul had been anchored in the Lord. It was all those decades she'd committed to church worship. Her brain had been trained. When she could not understand the world around her, when she feared everyone around her, she called out to her Lord, and her calling stirred something in me—and others.

God had planted the Lord's Prayer in my heart when Grandma and Granddad took me to church with them when I was a little girl, some forty years before I would need it for Grandma's healing. Closer to the time I would need this prayer, and Bible stories and classic hymns, for Grandma's healing, I was prompted by an experience in the hospital with Grandma. It happened when Grandma was scheduled for major surgery. There was a fifty-fifty chance she would survive it. On the eve of her surgery, I arrived at the hospital just in time. Grandma had been over-medicated and was so agitated she was fighting the staff. They were about to buckle thick leather strands around her wrists when I intervened. "Let me try something," I insisted. I grabbed a Bible from the nightstand next to her bed and began reading it. Instinctively, I knew that even when she was out of her mind, something deep inside her knew she had to quiet down when the Bible was being read. She had learned that as a little girl, and taught it to me in my youth.

It worked. Grandma dozed off, and so did Granddad. That surgery seemed to trigger her dementia, which was followed about a year after the operation by an official diagnosis of Alzheimer's. Occasionally violent and disoriented, more often quiet and vulnerable, Grandma became a test of my faith. She also became my Christ on the Cross, laying bare the frailty of our humanity and exposing the strength of our divinity. Jesus had come to teach unconditional love, and now it was making more sense to me. I loved Grandma despite her uncontrollable, sometimes violent behavior. I loved Granddad beyond his words and actions I believed to be wrong. They had taught me about religion and faith. This disease was teaching me about love.

Grandma had taught me much in my lifetime—how to cook, how to sew, how to love, and when to let go. Some of her old school lessons I turned upside down; and she never said so, but I think some of my responses to her lectures gave her something to think about. When I was in my late twenties she told me, "Men have to get a license to fish, or drive, or hunt. Make them get a license to be with you." I responded, "Grandma, I am not a sport or a plaything." She said I would learn. But in the end, she seemed to cheer my womanist ways, which her generation had not been afforded. When she spoke that old refrain, "Why buy the cow when you can get the milk free?" I shot back, "I am more than an animal, and I cannot be owned." That was the kind of relationship she and I enjoyed. I deeply admired her lifelong marriage, and felt deeply disappointed when I could not achieve it myself. But I also considered that I have been afforded freedoms and experiences my grandmother had not.

In the end, my brother was sure she admired my independence. He thought she had in some ways lived vicariously through me. Once, when I took Grandma and Granddad to a dinner theater with a couple of my friends who had once been married but now enjoyed life together as close friends, Grandma joked, "Can we have what they have?" And I was glad she acknowledged that her granddaughter was living in a whole new world.

When Grandma's Alzheimer's ushered us into a new dimension, it was old familiar songs that helped ground us. Some summer nights, Grandma and I sat on their front porch and sang her favorite hymns: "At the Cross," "Power in the Blood," and "Keep Me Near the Cross," to name a few.

I attended six weeks of workshops for Alzheimer's caregivers at the Veterans Affairs hospital and found the meditation tools, pep talks, shared stories, and listings of available resources extremely helpful. Yet living with Alzheimer's day-to-day I learned even more. I learned the value of patience. Learned what the Bible means when it says love is long-suffering. I learned a lot from Granddad's determination to keep his wife home. When Grandma's violent spells got so bad I worried she might push him down the stairs to his death, he still would not concede.

"I'd be lonesome without her," he said sadly.

All the turmoil and the tests we were experiencing together struck down a lot of my old judgments about my grandparents, especially Granddad. I'd considered him verbally abusive. Had blamed his controlling behavior for Grandma's mental deterioration. From the early stages of her dementia, I would confront him about his tone of voice with her. "That tone of voice rattles her," I scolded. "It rattles me!" One Sunday morning, on our way to church, Granddad, seated up front in the passenger's seat, ranted and raved bitterly. Grandma's response from the back was, "Go ahead and get it all out. Cleanse yourself out." In that moment, I considered that all those years I heard fussing, she'd heard a man crying like a baby.

She had been a nurse, and she knew the meaning of tears better than I did. Even with Alzheimer's, Grandma experienced incredible moments of lucidity when she would drop me a pearl of wisdom. "Let the Lord fight your battles," she said, seemingly out-the-blue in church one morning. We were standing, singing and clapping in praise, and she turned to me with that bit of peace. I looked at her and smiled. I was going through a divorce, which I had not discussed with her. Another time, we were having dinner at their dining room table and she turned to me and said, "Ray-Ray, don't let anybody intimidate you. I don't care how much money they have, or what position they got on the job. You are just as good as anybody else."

Within moments she was back in her private world, a sort of dazed look on her face. One time after work I was sitting on a stool in the kitchen talking to Granddad about a conflict at work. Granddad was stirring pots on the stove, and Grandma was sweeping the floor. I didn't think she was paying attention to what I was saying until she turned to me and said, "Raise your skirt hem a little, just a little." I said, "Huh?" And she added, "Your boss is a man, isn't he? Raise the hem on your skirt a little." Granddad and I burst out laughing. I had only known Grandma as the staunch deaconess who had chided me for wearing super-tight or see-through pants.

According to her doctor, Grandma's brain cells were like a light switch with a faulty cord. Sometimes the connectors worked and she could understand and articulate. I treasured those rare moments.

In the end, I was grateful for what I had learned for Grandma and from her. I had learned the songs and prayers that would soothe her in her final years. I had learned from her life skills and insights that could comfort me the rest of my life. Most importantly, through this experience I learned the power of prayer. When I told a dear friend about this experience, she suggested that the prayers had also summoned angels into the house. She shared a similar experience she'd had repeating Hail Mary prayers over herself, feeling certain pains dissipate.

Grandma died in 2016 at ninety-seven years old. As my family recovered from this, I had time to reflect on the lessons. One Sunday morning I was on my way to pick up Granddad for church and heard the song, "My Soul Has Been Anchored in the Lord," on the radio, and my heart smiled. During church that morning, a surprise guest emerged with his saxophone and played that song. The irony compelled further consideration. Anchored in the Lord? That's got to mean more than being anchored in churchgoing. I considered that being anchored in the Lord is being anchored in Love because Jesus Christ's great commission was to teach humanity to love and forgive. Thanks to what I had to give and what I received caring for Grandma, I am better anchored in love to survive life's inevitable storms.

REVELATIONS
Loretta Anne Woodward Veney

For more than thirty years, it was a tradition for our family to journey together to the Kennedy Center to see the Alvin Ailey American Dance company. We never missed a year. My mom, Doris, was always the organizer. She kept count of how many family members would be going, purchased the tickets months in advance, and even allowed those on a budget to save up to pay her back on the day of the performance. Mom's favorite Ailey dance was "Revelations," and we always bought tickets to attend the performance that featured that dance.

In addition to Mom and me, other family members attending included my grandmother Alberta, my aunt Diane, and my sister Renee, and four or five cousins always joined us when they were available. The informal rules required those attending to dress up for the event. We all looked forward to this annual family tradition, but none of us as much as my Mom. For her, seeing the Alvin Ailey dancers was nearly a religious experience.

"Revelations" is Alvin Ailey's signature dance and has been since it premiered in 1960. It is performed to some of the most moving spirituals ever written, including "I've Been 'Buked and Scorned," and "Wade in the Water." The costumes worn by the dancers are spectacular and colorful, swirling as the dancers spin across the floor. The choreography and music are so mesmerizing; the nearly thirty-minute performance turns the concert hall into a church and your seat into a pew. My mom usually always cried during the dance, and she wasn't alone, as many others in the audience were moved to tears as well, simply because of the pure beauty of the dance.

Over the three decades that our family saw Alvin Ailey each year, family attendance changed dramatically. My grandmother and Aunt Diane both died of colon cancer, my cousins were busy with careers and family, and my niece and sister were now living in California. Yet even after Mom was diagnosed with dementia in 2006, she and I continued to attend the Alvin Ailey performance. Mom enjoyed the shows as she always had. We just kept a closer eye on her in the crowd before and after the performance.

The evening that changed everything, I had purchased front row tickets for me and Mom to be as close to the stage as possible, hoping that would ensure Mom would recall her favorite performance. That evening I had helped Mom dress in her favorite burgundy suit with a green-and-burgundy-flowered blouse and her fancy black shoes. She looked beautiful. I thought sure she'd remember the Kennedy Center, but when we entered the huge concert hall, Mom asked, "We haven't been here before, have we?" I assured her that we had been coming to this event for many years, and she said, "Oh."

Almost as soon as the performance began, I knew bringing Mom had been a mistake. Even in the darkened hall I could see the blank stare in Mom's eyes, and she asked, "Where are we?" She watched the dancers glide across the floor, but she clearly couldn't make sense of what was happening. My stomach clenched, and I felt sick. Even though Mom looked confused, she seemed content enough, but I was worried that she'd eventually get frightened by the loud music and scream out that she wanted to go home. Thankfully she didn't. As the performance progressed, Mom clapped at the end of each dance, but she still had no idea what was happening or where she was. In previous years, she was always on the edge of her seat watching every move, but this time she stared straight ahead with her hands folded in her lap.

In spite of all that, I was sure she'd "come alive" when "Revelations" unfolded onstage. But she didn't. As the music started, she sat unmoving and unfazed. I whispered to her, "This is your favorite dance." She said, "Uh huh," clearly not understanding what I meant. I panicked. Why wasn't she remembering her favorite dance of all time? I started to silently cry because I was having a revelation of my own. I never thought I'd see the day when Mom didn't remember her favorite dance, yet that day had come. I was devastated and held her hand for the last ten minutes or so of "Revelations." I cried even harder at the end of the dance because I knew I had seen it for the last time with Mom. I wondered when she'd eventually no longer recognize me.

When the performance was over, I was emotionally drained. I had spent almost $300 on an event that Mom had no idea we attended. As we always did, we headed to the restroom before heading home. We got in the long line, and Mom stared down at the program in her hands. She read the title out loud, "The Alvin Ailey Dancers." Then she said, "You always used to take me to see this show, why don't you take me anymore?" I tried to quietly explain that we had just seen the show, and then she shot back loudly, "That is my favorite dance troupe! I would KNOW if I had just seen it." Other women in the restroom line started to fidget and look around awkwardly. Then Mom turned and ran from me, which she'd never done before! My leg was in a cast at the time and I couldn't chase her, so a woman who had been in line ran to retrieve Mom for me. I felt a pain in my heart I'd never felt before. Life as we knew and loved it really had ended.

Mom had loved dance her entire life, and now she had no idea what it was or what it had meant to her. I held Mom by the shoulders and took her to a stairwell so we could be alone and explained to her that we had just seen the show and that she was holding the program in her hand. Sobbing, she said, "You spent all that money on these tickets, and I can't even remember." I told her it was okay, and that I loved her. She said she loved me too, and I hugged her as tightly as I could because I wanted to make it all better, just as she had done so many times for me when I was a child. We held hands and slowly walked back to the restroom to wait our turn.

Once back in line, I started to explain to her the dances that had been performed, and she listened intently. Her eyes locked on mine as I began to explain, and she nodded as if she was actually following what I was saying. I had left out an important detail of one of the dances, and a woman behind us said, "Don't forget to tell her about . . . " And she filled in some of the blanks for me. I was relieved that someone understood what I was trying to do for Mom now that her brain no longer worked the way it used to. Standing in that restroom, I was devastated that this would be the last time my mother and I would share this cultural ritual, but I also felt loved, encouraged, and supported, by the other women in line in the ladies' room, who understood what I was going through.

I haven't been to see the Alvin Ailey dancers since that night. I don't think I can return and watch "Revelations" again without my mom and not feel overwhelmed by the grief of what we have lost. I hope to be able to go again at some point, maybe with my grand-daughter who is now six years old, so that she and I can start a new family tradition. I think Mom would be proud if I did that, but I know that emotionally it's still a few years away for me. Dementia robs families of everything, starting with their joy and traditions, but it can't take away the love shared between family members. The last thing Mom said to me when we got home that night was "Thank you for always taking care of me." Since then we've discovered other new traditions to share, and it doesn't matter if Mom only remembers the experience for just one second, or not at all. Every day we are still together is a revelation.

ALL THAT REMAINS

INTRODUCTION

The disease appears to take everything. Everything, that is, that we value most. *Speech*, although body language is the most precise indicator of what we feel and think. Our words are so often throbbing with mixed, muddled emotions, and varied intent. *Memory*, even as we know that our memories are subjective, unreliable; as often as not the manifestation of wish-fulfillment or denial. Alzheimer's, the most common form of dementia, eventually will take it all—*movement, thought, bodily functions.* The brain, the god of intelligence, cognition, and wisdom, becomes a ruin, a desolate region, incapable of harvesting the kind of thoughts that affirm, measure, and define what we think of as life.

But before the end, in the long strange journey to the end, there is much that remains. If our brain empowers us with resolve and resilience, our hearts are the Petri dish for the soul we cannot see but only verify by the yearnings unbidden and unimagined that startle and salvage us. The brain is how we live; the heart is in the most metaphorical and figurative sense why we live. How else to explain that the deserted and desert-like brain recedes, and the heart and soul begin to blossom amidst the bleakness and despair of dementia?

"All that remains" is an assertion rather than a qualification, a confirmation announcing the persistent presence of all that does, somehow, remain. Acceptance remains, because dementia provides no oxygen for denial. The present moment remains, overlooked, brushed aside, until the present moment is literally the last possession of the dementia-mind. Laughter remains, God's reward for not giving up. Conversation too, pieced together like puzzles that make all the sense the moment requires. These and even more are *all that remain.*

THE LAST CONVERSATION
Bari Diane Adelman

My darling eighty-eight-year-old mother has had progressive dementia for a decade. She has lost her sight, hearing, and speech, and I miss
her terribly. I miss her warmth, her wisdom, her wit.

Shortly before Mom lost her ability to speak, we had an important conversation.

The chat was truncated as a result of Mom's limited cognitive
abilities. Speaking coherently had grown increasingly difficult for
her, and I was terrified that our ability to have any future dialogue
was shrinking. Instinct was telling me this might be one of the last
conversations we would ever have, and though it was rather basic, I
felt an urge to record it.

The conversation took place while we were browsing through a
family photo album. Mom kept asking me who the "strangers" in
the photos were—strangers who included her husband, children, and
grandchildren.

Mom turned to me and said, "Bari, something terrible is happening to me. This shouldn't happen to a person."

"You're right," I answered.

"I don't want to be a burden," she said.

I turned and looked her in the eye. "You're not."

"Where do I live? Who takes care of me?"

"You live in a wonderful assisted living facility, where you and
Dad share an apartment."

"But I don't want to be a burden to him," she insisted.

"You're not, Mom. Dad loves you and wants to be there with you.

And please don't worry—there are lots of people who help Dad. They serve you three meals a day and do all the laundry and chores."

"But I don't want to be a burden," she insisted.

"Dad loves you, Mom. We all love you. This is what families do. We take care of each other."

The words were simple, but for years now, I have turned to them many times over. They sustain me. They fill a void.

"I don't want to be a burden." This was the mantra of Mom's life. She prided herself on being strong, independent, and self-sufficient. Highly educated, Mom had successfully combined career and motherhood well before that was fashionable, first as a high school teacher, then school librarian, and ultimately college advisor. She wanted to add value to the world, not be a drain. With these words, Mom was telling me she feared her worst nightmare was befalling her.

Even more significantly, this was the one and only time Mom acknowledged to me that she knew something was wrong with her. Until then, she had been either unable or unwilling to do so. I had tried to initiate gentle conversation about her decline, several times in fact, but Mom always deflected the conversation, and I felt I had to honor what was denial or willful ignorance on her part—though perhaps it was a complete lack of awareness.

This was the first time since Mom had gotten sick that she seemed able to confront the fact that something terrible was happening to her. Something she didn't understand but despaired of. She had seen this happen to her own mother and had lived with the fear it would happen to her. Here was Mom, for the very first time, sharing her fear and pain with me. There was urgency in her voice and tone as she reached out with the only words she could find. I felt her despair.

But how to respond? In the few seconds available to come up with a reply, my subconscious mind kicked in instinctively. I desperately wanted to validate Mom's feelings and soothe her soul. I couldn't find adequate words but tried to assure her I was there for her and let her know that we, her family, didn't feel it was a burden to care for her. I know the love and intention behind my words were pure. And I believe she could feel that.

So many years have passed since that moment. I visit Mom at her nursing home three times a week. I hug her, kiss her cheek, and whisper "I love you" in her ear each and every time. But I have lost my mother.

When my pain is at its most raw, my memory of that last conversation sustains me. I am grateful I documented Mom's words and take comfort in knowing that in those few moments, I did everything I could to offer her a sense of relief and calm. I want her to be at peace. To know how much she was, and is, appreciated and loved. That she could never be a burden.

DEVIL'S ALLEY
TINA JENKINS BELL

I was trapped in a devil's alley, a place without exits or windows, after losing my brother Champ to idiopathic pulmonary fibrosis (IPF) and seeing Mama's will to fight her dementia bottom out.

It was 5:00 on a Saturday morning. Every light was on in my home, except for the bedrooms where my boys slept, completely oblivious to my desperation. Mama's neighbor, Ms. Tolliver, had called to alert us Mama was "in the wind" again and had apparently boarded a Western Avenue bus in front of her building around 4:00 a.m.

My husband, Earl, worried aloud about me scouring Chicago streets in search of my mother before sunrise, but he knew I needed to act. Mama's doctor was aware of her tendency to flee and advised us to institutionalize her for her good . . . and ours.

"She needs twenty-four-hour nursing care. Frankly, when I'm her age, I've directed my children to put me in a home and forget I'm there. Dementia ravages the person who has it and their caretakers, too," Dr. Assad had said.

I dressed quickly and went to my Jeep to warm the engine. The sky emptied snow from above, and snowflakes cartwheeled across the car's hood. Meanwhile, I waited for my sister Cynthia, who lived with us after being displaced from a long-time job, and wondered why God hadn't noticed I'd reached my limit.

Minutes later, Cynthia emerged, holding a cup in one hand and a set of keys in the other. She flopped in the passenger's seat.

"Damn, when is this going to end?"

I blew warm air into my bare hands before putting gloves on and maneuvering the car into drive. "I don't know."

We both sighed as an apprehensive quiet permeated the car. I focused on the road, watching landmarks, from St. Rita High School just past 79th Street to Gage Park's Gothic-style fieldhouse, glide by while Cynthia glanced out of the passenger's window. "You think we might not find her this time?"

"Nope," I said. "We'll find her, hopefully before the police." From the side of my eye, I saw Cynthia nod. Even with a seatbelt on, her shoulders drooped. She looked as tired as I felt. Neither of us had been getting much sleep since Champ's death, which was devastating. He was Mama's only son and the closest resemblance to the husband she'd lost forty-six years prior when I was just three months old. She loved him to no end, making him our responsibility to protect. But none of us could beat IPF, so Mama gave in to a world where her beloveds— Champ, her mother, her grandfather, and my dad—still lived.

Before Mama's shift from the present, she was a reader and letter writer with a strong head for managing finances. When she casually asked me one day to balance her checkbook, I was flabbergasted. She prided herself in doing most things on her own, particularly "money" things. Then, a careful survey revealed she'd overpaid Visa by $5,000. Checks began to bounce shortly after that. Later, I would get a call from the office manager at Mama's former apartment building. She hadn't paid her rent.

"You *are* talking about Helen Jenkins," I checked.

"I'm talking about Helen," Mrs. Davis said, as her usual crisp voice began to mellow. "It's not her fault. She was embarrassed to admit con artists picked her up at the Metro Grocery Store and . . . well, just ask her."

I ripped out a check for $500 and handed it to Ms. Davis. "I got this."

"I know you do, honey. Helen is lucky to have y'all. God bless, okay?" I nodded and took the elevator to Mama's fifth floor apartment, where she told me the rest of the story.

"They needed me to go the currency exchange to get some more

money. But I had to cash my check and give them my money first."
Mama's eyes enlarged and teared with recognition behind her black-
rimmed glasses. "I don't know what I was thinking."

I concurred. Mama didn't usually trust anyone, even her own
children. She'd have never gotten into the car with strangers, but
I was her child and couldn't admonish her. I empathized instead.
"Those rat bastards had better be sure I don't catch their asses."

This made her happy. Though we were cultured, she brought us
up with Marine mentalities. We'd kick behinds for family.

Then out of nowhere came this tiny voice I never would have
associated with my mom. "Don't let them put me away, like they did
my mama."

My grandmother had been institutionalized in the notorious
Mississippi State Hospital for the Insane when my mother was ten
years old. Traumatized by the experience, Mama made us promise
to protect her independence, no matter what. No nursing homes. No
hospitals for seniors with issues. We tried to comply, so after the con
artist incident, we'd moved her to a senior citizen apartment building
on 45th and Western, closer to my home.

Proximity didn't matter; Mama easily circumvented our monitoring efforts when a goal pressed her like the one that led her to rise at
4:00 a.m. to catch a bus.

Cynthia and I scrutinized buses and sidewalks for four hours
before returning to Mama's apartment. We found her cooking a
Kwanzaa dinner for Champ. It was March; Champ had been gone
for a month; and Kwanzaa follows Christmas.

"I needed a few things to complete Champ's dinner," she said
after being bombarded with our questions about her whereabouts.

Numb, Cynthia and I glanced at each other; our eyes became
wells of unfallen tears as we struggled once more with nudging
Mama from her demented state back into reality and forcing her to
relive her boy's death. At least for that day, we decided to quell our
own grief and postpone another round of the same heartbreak for
Mama.

Playing along, Cynthia said, "Are those turnip greens I smell?"

With a hand on her hip and the other stirring something in a tall pot, Mama smiled,

"Yes. Champ's favorite."

I joined the charade. "Well, they may be Champ's favorite, but I love them, too. Where's the Tupperware?"

Behind us, the sun, a ball of yellow, polished silver, shone through Mama's floor-to-ceiling windows, but neither Cynthia nor I could bask in it. Instead, we watched Mama move purposefully in her kitchen, where she'd always found comfort, cooking turkey, greens, black-eyed peas, macaroni and cheese, dinner rolls, and sweet potato pies. We had completed our mission. Mama was home, happy and safe for now. Still, there were crooks and turns in the devil's alley, and though Mama was where we could see her today, the chase could very well be on again tomorrow.

MOTHER'S MEMORIES
DANIELLE BELTON

Who is the keeper of your mother's memories when she can't remember them?

Now, are you someone I'm supposed to know?

She's nice enough on the phone. Pleasant, even. So pleasant that it could be normal if you wanted to pretend. But then, she's always been nice, always liked to talk, even if she had nothing to say. This was no different, although these days she has good days and bad days. Before my father put her on the phone, I asked if she was in a good mood. Today was one of the good days, he said, so he gave my mother the phone, and there she was.

Just happy to be here. Laughing at nothing.

"Hi, Mommy," I said, like I used to say it when I was little. High-pitched and chipper. Youthful and hopeful.

"Hi, Mommy," she chirped back to me, parroting my tone.

That wasn't the right response. My heart fell. It was a "good" day, but she'd gotten worse. Just a few months ago, she could still recognize my voice, sometimes. But now the memory of my voice, of me, was finally gone.

"So you're one of the people I'm supposed to know?" she said, chuckling.

"This is Danielle," I said.

"Danielle," she repeated to me, as if she were thinking about it.

"Your daughter," I said.

Our conversation was brief. She laughed, a lot, at nothing in particular. When I told her work was good, she laughed. When I told I was in good health and the weather was nice, she laughed. She asked me where I was, and I told her Washington, DC; she laughed.

"Oh," she said, laughing. "Well, I'm sure you're busy, and I don't want to keep you."

My mother is still here with us, but her mind left us long ago. Dementia has robbed her of her memories and personality, leaving behind a woman who looks exactly like my mother and sounds exactly like my mother but is no longer my mother. She's also no longer my father's wife, her mother's daughter, a sister to her many siblings, a niece to her surviving aunt and uncle, a grandmother to her only grandchild, or any of the things that made her just her, that made her Deloris—or, as her family called her, Babyray, the person we all loved.

It's a testament to how good she was as a mother, wife, daughter, sister, niece, grandmother, and friend that everyone still calls, everyone still visits, everyone still wants to see her even though she couldn't care less who we all are. My father and sisters look after her back in St. Louis while I'm just a voice on a phone, hiding from everything.

My father tells me, repeatedly, to live my life because that's what he wants, that's what she would have wanted if she were still herself. He has been telling me this since 2009, when I left home for the second time in my life to move to DC. Even though she wasn't sick then, I felt bad about leaving my parents because they were getting older. I wanted to spend as much time with them as I could. I wanted to take care of them. But there also wasn't any work for me as a writer in St. Louis.

So I left.

When my friend Toya passed away almost two years ago from colon cancer, the thing I lamented the most was that when she went, she took all her memories with her. All the things that made her who she was were lost to the world. It's the same with my mother, only she lives on, oblivious to what she's lost, and to what she continues to lose every day.

Who is the keeper of your mother's memories when she can't remember them?

My mother comes to me in my dreams. In the dreams she is always leaving me, us, our family, and I'm angry with her because she is cold and unforgiving. But at least in the dreams she is herself. Not the side of her that I liked, but she is "Deloris." In the last dream I had about her, she was divorcing my father, to whom she's been married for more than forty years. She was youthful-looking, clad in a stylish gold dress, and her curly hair was immaculately laid. She looked beautiful—cold and distant, but beautiful. And in the dream, she yelled at me the way she used to when I was a teenager, when we used to get into these terrible fights where she would badger me until I was in tears, utterly destroyed. In the dream, I told her how angry I was at her for leaving us, but it made no difference. She was still going.

I honestly would have preferred a world where my mother still possessed her mind, even if it was only the side of her that I didn't like. I wish she had just abandoned all of us like in my dream because the greatest tragedy of losing her, of dementia, is that she is lost to herself. If she'd just been like how she was in my dream, she'd still be Deloris and all the things that made her her.

Deloris, who liked arguing politics and was once labeled a "militant" parent because she pushed so hard for the better education of black children in her neighborhood.

Deloris, who was talkative, outgoing, and friendly, but at her core, still a shy Southern girl from Arkansas.

Deloris, who liked to be number one in your heart even as she was pissing you off.

Deloris, who never said a curse word but whose favorite comedian was Richard Pryor and who loved the raunchiest, dirtiest blues music known to mankind.

Deloris, who wore high heels everywhere and wore makeup to everything, who was a voracious reader and thinker, who loved children, holidays, pecans, and shopping malls, who talked to everyone as if they were her best friend even if she had no idea who they were.

Today, to my mother, my sisters and I are kind strangers. Our father is "that guy." Her grandson is some "handsome young boy."

She forgets to call her mother, who is dealing with the horror and indignity of having your own child forget you while you're still living. My sisters, father, and I try to find humor where we can. We've all come to accept what has become of her in our own ways. Mother's Day is still Mother's Day, even if she's forgotten that she was a mother. We remember for her. Remind her. Love her. We are the keepers of her memories now. We're the ones who tell her story.

We're the ones who celebrate her while she's still here, even though she's gone.

THE OTHER SIDE OF HERE

An Excerpt from *The Long Hello*

CATHIE BORRIE

Every day I sit with my mother and watch the sea.

There's a row of birds perched on an errant log—cormorant, cormorant, seagull, heron. Crow.

"Cathie, sometimes I drift off for ten minutes and I don't know where I've gone."

"Does that bother you, Mum?"

"No, it doesn't. Are you my daughter?"

We watch frantic wing-flitting at her bird feeder. Chickadees, starlings, sparrows. A house finch, brown-striped.

"Cath, I think it's a finch, it's only . . . oh—a finch a finch a finch! Are they trying to tell you they aren't in there? What are they trying to say?"

"To say . . . ? I don't know."

"I think there's something, they're trying to get something across, aren't they, love?"

* * *

I tell people I'm still working and making money but I'm not. Try to ignore the tightness in my chest from having to move so slowly when I like moving fast, and the creeping sense of captivity that sits heavy in my gut.

My mother sits on her couch with her eyes closed.

"Would you like to have a little rest?"

"Okay, dear. But where are you going to sit? And then you're going to go away with Dad, aren't you, and I'll be all alone."

"I never go away with Dad."

"Oh, that's good."

"You seem so tired . . . are you giving up?"

"No, I don't give up. I don't know how to do it."

"Neither do I."

I draw the curtains.

"How was your day?"

"It's very hard for me to tell you because when you say, 'How have you been today, Mum?' I try to think, and I can't think of anything. I don't know what I did this morning, I have no idea."

"Oh. Maybe a better question would be—how are you right now?"

"Well, I'm fine, just fine. Yes, it's a good, a better question to come for me."

"You look like a little porcelain doll lying there."

"Does it, does it look just like china?"

"Yes, just perfect."

"Well, that's good. Somebody's got to be perfect."

* * *

As soon as I'm home I call to say good night.

"Hi Mum, it's Cath. What are you doing?"

"I'm waiting for you. . . . I'm just here waiting for you."

"But I just got home. I was just over there."

"Over here?"

"Yes . . . never mind. I'll call first thing in the morning, okay?"

"Where are you? I couldn't find you."

"I'm home, I'm at my home. I'm fine."

"I thought I'd left you in the living room, all alone."

I drink two glasses of my favorite red wine, eat two bars of dark chocolate, swallow one and a half sleeping pills, and sink down into nothing. I crawl into bed in my clothes, pull the radio up beside me, and tune in my favorite all-night talk show. Tonight's program features government conspiracies, CIA subterfuge, contrail theory, alien abductions. The window is wide open, my bedroom is freezing. I wrap the sheet around my face, a shroud. As far as my mind can see there is nothing.

Everywhere.

My new favorite thing.

* * *

When my mother can't get in and out of the bath anymore, I wear a green garbage bag over my clothes and help her in the shower. We're both embarrassed.

"I don't mind, Mum. You gave me lots of baths when I was a baby."

"I'm not a baby."

"I didn't mean . . ."

I can't get the room warm enough, the water temperature right. She shivers, her thin, dry skin flaking off on the towel. I feel sick.

"Love, do be careful. Don't let me fall!"

"I'm sorry, I'm sorry."

When we can't manage showers anymore she goes to the Seniors' Day Centre for her weekly bath and hair wash in a bright, heated room. There's a towel warmer, lavender-scented suds, kind staff, a yellow rubber duck.

Once a month we visit her doctor for advice, prescriptions, and for the kind words she makes sure my mother hears during every visit.

"You're doing so well."

"I know, I'm much better."

"Yes, you are. I just want to listen to your chest today."

"Oh yeah, you and all the other boys."

"Good one! I know you had some trouble with that pill I gave you and I'd like to try another one."

"I just can't remember things. My mind, it's all mixed up."

"Mrs. B., Parkinson's does that in some people, so I'm hoping this drug will help with that. I'm really very impressed with how you're doing."

My mother beams and for the rest of the day she goes over and over what the doctor has told her.

"Did you hear what she said? She thinks I'm doing really well and I am, you know. I'm better every day."

"She's really pleased with you."

"Do you really think so? Oh my."

When she no longer remembers the visits, I tell her what the doctor has said.

"She said she was really pleased with you and that you are doing a really good job."

"And then what did I say?"

"You told her that you were trying very hard."

"I did? Well, that sounds silly."

"Um, oh, and then you thanked her for her kindness and for being such a good doctor."

"Oh, that's better. Yes, I like that better."

When we get home, I put on the kettle.

"Are you happy?"

"Yes."

"How happy?"

"I'm very happy."

"Because?"

"Because I have no faith in anyone."

I start to close the blinds.

"Leave the curtains open so I can see the birds."

"How does one look after a bird?"

"Unless it's very tame, you can't. You know, I'm twice bitten and three times shy and I can't remember. Listen—a bird!"

"What are the birds saying?"

"They're chirping."

"In a language?"

"In their language. In an upside-down language."

* * *

Love? How do I get home or when I get home how do I get home?"

"Mum, you are home, see all your things around you?"

"These are my things? How did they get here? I think that girl, she was the one I found most interesting but sometimes I think she employed too much use of the wind."

"Who? Who was that?"

"Who? You're a regular customer and I'm the one that rushes in, all eyes. This is my home? Do I own it?"

"Yes, you own it and you'll always be able to stay here."

"Good, because I never want to leave here. Getting them unscrambled is an important thing—you go seven, eight, nine, which means you're pretty strong which is a good thing. And the birds, that's what they were screaming about, these little ones this morning."

"What were they saying?"

"They said, 'Stay little one, stay.' And I said, 'Okay, okay.'"

"That should settle it."

I make tea.

"Tea is a more pleasant drink. It just seems to sort of go down and settle things."

"You're my favorite person in the world."

"Favorite amongst the constipated you mean."

"How was your day?"

"Today I was down at the horse barn. It came with lots of blessings."

"Oh my . . . I love listening to you talk."

"You love what?"

"Listening to you talk."

"Oh. I thought I heard you say, I love looking into your voice."

"I love that, too."

WHAT HAPPENED TO BRAD?

An Excerpt from *Minding Our Elders:*
Caregivers Share Their Personal Stories

CAROL BRADLEY BURSACK

Dad was agitated. I could tell by his jerky movements, his flushed skin. He was perched on the edge of his lift chair, shuffling though a pile of papers on his knees, some of which were spilling onto the floor. A table on his left was covered with sticky folders and curled, spotted business papers. Three overstuffed briefcases and a file gaped open; more papers crouched under the sink and huddled under his chair. Juice-soaked business cards stuck to the wheeled table on his right, joined by his candy basket, call-light, tissues, and boom box. He looked up hopefully as I walked into his room.

"Good. There you are," he said. "I need you to . . . to . . . take some, uh, some, dic . . . oh . . . oh . . . some dictation."

I caught a sigh before it escaped and replaced it with a smile and breezy attitude, as I kissed him hello.

"Sure. I can do that anytime. How are you?"

His eyes were red and unfocused, the look of his very delusional phase—as opposed to his somewhat delusional phase. My mission was to tame the tigers in his brain, so he can relax for a time.

"What I need is a list. The city commissioners. A list of them because of the elephants. I need you to write a . . . oh, a . . . a . . . you know what I need, just write a . . . a . . . pro . . . pro—"

"A proposal?" I ask. "Sure, I can write a proposal. You want the commissioners to get an elephant for the city?"

"We've been working on it," he answered. "But no! Not the . . .

not the commissioners, but I've been working on . . . I've been asked . . . they've asked me to get an elephant and be a part . . ."

My brain searched for answers as it tried to separate the scrambled images Dad was relating. I got out the yellow legal pad he keeps by his chair and began taking dictation. His fingers are numb, and his eyes, ears, and brain are marginal, but tools for his work he must have.

"We are getting a new zoo, which is no longer a city project, but there is a zoo board. I'll bet you're working with *them* to bring in an elephant," I said. I was beginning to feel the effect of endorphins, a feeling that I could go the distance this time. I wrote: *elephant*.

But then.

"And that Catholic prayer . . . the one that repeats . . . repeats . . . Mary . . . something, bring me that. I need that."

Considering our Presbyterian heritage, that was an unusual request, but, after six years of this, I am rarely surprised.

"Oh, you mean the Hail Mary?" I ask. "Hail Mary, full of grace? The one they say for the rosary?"

"Yes! Yes!" he answered, looking at me as if I truly had lost my mind this time. "Yes, why do you ask?" he said.

"Sure," I said, grateful for the Catholic friends of my childhood, and my dear Catholic friend Jane, who taught me that prayer. Dad had raised exotic ants between the windows, kept bees (who wintered in our garage), dug for fossils, and scoped out the planets. In context, his need to bring an elephant to Fargo, or to have the words to a Catholic prayer, were mundane.

I wrote: *Hail Mary*.

"And the names of the commissioners, and their phone numbers and the addresses and where to put the elephant," he said.

I wrote: *list commissioners*.

"Okay," I said. "I'll have the zoo board contact you about the elephant, type up the Hail Mary, and get a list of commissioners. Will that do it?"

"I think so. Yes, good. Yes, that should be good," he said.

His color improved, the agitation slowly drained away. My jaw relaxed, and I breathed more easily as I realized that today I'd won. Just for today, I had quieted the chaos.

How to proceed in filling his needs for tomorrow? The Hail Mary, no problem, I know it and can type it out. The commissioners, no problem. In fact, I'll get him the meeting notes off the Internet.

But the elephant and the zoo. A little challenge. I'll have to write a letter from the zoo to Dad, thanking him for his interest, and inviting him to help them in the future when they are ready to bring in the elephant. Shouldn't be too bad. Easier than the letter from the military thanking him for wanting to be an officer, or any of several letters from our mayor. I really should let Mr. Furness know about the letters he's written Dad. Some other time.

Dad's given name was Clarence, but he was always known as Brad. He was a retired city employee, growing old, a bit confused, but still Brad. Fluid had begun to build up in the scar tissue left behind from a closed head injury sustained during maneuvers in World War II. Dad, the skinny, fair fellow whose ancestors thrived in cloudy England, collapsed while training in the Mojave Desert, smacking his head against desert rock. He was in a coma for weeks, then spent months in rehabilitation, learning to walk and talk. He fought through hell to lead a normal life, working, fathering two more children, earning a college degree, holding the position of supervising sanitarian for the city of Fargo.

But as he grew older the injury began to haunt him. His waterlogged thinking would grow worse if he didn't have a shunt put in his brain to channel off the fluid. Specialists recommended the operation.

Surgery day. As they wheeled him away, Dad forced a smile, thumb and forefinger creating a circle signaling "okay."

Hours later, we faced a sleepy man. We were filled with hope.

Days later we came to realize Brad had gone to sleep on that operating table and Clarence had awakened, with a voice firmly implanted in his head, a voice we came to call Herman. My dad, as I knew him, was dead. We were filled with despair.

Our family has soldiered on. Since that time, I've created the degrees he thinks he's earned, designed the awards he thinks he's received, written the letters he thinks are coming. One morning, blood pressure and pulse barely there, he's Rip Van Winkle. Another morning, bright-eyed and mischievous, he's Dennis the Menace. He can be a great musician, a military officer, a doctor, lawyer, or president of the United States. A few loyal friends still struggle to visit him, but the visits can be so distressing that most stay away. Clarence is a bit frightening, and they want to remember Brad.

Dad was born prematurely in 1917; he's been hospitalized for pneumonia twice, and nearly died from a penicillin reaction. He survived a closed head injury to claim the life God promised him. So, what are a few elephants? I'll see what I can do.

FEAR AND LAUGHING
LISA FRIEDMAN

Our worst fear has recently come to pass: the dementia ward of the veterans' home where my father had been living transferred him to a psychiatric hospital. But when I met my mother there on the day they brought him over, I wasn't really surprised to see her waving from across the hall with a big smile on her face, about to laugh. We're a family of laughers. We laugh when we're happy, when we're angry, and, most of all, when we're frightened.

"That's him," she said, chortling and pointing to the ambulance in the bay. "He just arrived, and he's mad as a wet hen. But the ambulance driver said he didn't slug anyone, so that's an improvement."

They wheeled my father up. "Hi, Dad." I touched his hand, which was locked down under a thick restraining belt. His sweat pants were stained with food; the socks on his feet twisted and wrong. He looked at me through the blue eyes I've been looking into for forty-nine years. I smiled at him and winked. He winked back. He is seventy-five and in perfect health if you don't count his brain. He's had dementia for a few years, but things got worse after an adverse drug reaction.

They pulled the gurney away. "We'll meet you inside!" I yelled. My father craned his neck and answered: "Two. Four. Seventeen!"

My mother and I followed someone into the admitting office to do the paperwork. "We brought his medical records," I told the nurse, reaching across the desk to where my mother sat, stalwart. I wiggled my fingers for the papers, but my mother only glared at me.

"Mom. Pass me the records."

She shook her head.

The nurse moved away, ostensibly to retrieve a form. I leaned toward my mother. "What are you doing?"

My mother gripped her purse with two hands. "I don't want them to have a bad impression of your father," she said. I reached for her purse. She held tight. I pulled.

"We probably shouldn't have an altercation," I said, pausing. "It might look bad."

My mother smiled. Look bad? We were in a mental hospital. Who cared? We both began to laugh, gently at first, and then with increasing gusto. By the time the nurse returned, it took all of our shared strength to stop.

The nurse handed us an information sheet. "This is the number of the telephone on the ward," she said, pointing with her pencil. "Call this number anytime and ask to speak with your husband," she explained, looking kindly at my mother.

Later we sat with my father on the ward, trying not to cry. For months, professionals had been saying that he'd probably need to go to the psychiatric hospital. But we'd closed our minds to that possibility. My mother declared she would not survive it. And now here we were.

We sat on either side of him, distracting ourselves with his food tray. I cut up the chicken and put the loaded fork into my father's hand. My leg bounced off his—something was there.
"There's something in Dad's pocket," I informed my mother. "Put your hand in there and pull it out, will you?"

She crossed her eyes. "I'm not doing it. You do it."

I held my breath and reached in—and then extracted a brightly colored, stuffed bowling pin. I held it up and met my mother's disbelieving stare. That did it; we collapsed into gales of wrenching laughter again, hiding behind our hands and lowering our heads into our collars.

"Stop," my mother begged with her eyes flooding tears. "Stop, or they won't let us out!"

I got up and walked away, wiping my eyes. I imagined I looked like every other visitor, splotchy with emotion and bereavement. When I regained my composure, I returned to the table. My mother had stepped into the bathroom; my father was eating his napkin.

Soon it was time to leave him there. As we waited to be escorted through the double-locked doors, the hall phone began to ring. A woman appeared wearing a long purple sweater and opera-length pearls. She picked up the phone and began to speak gibberish with a Slavic accent. She chattered, listened, and then hung up. As she walked away, we saw that she was naked from the waist down.

My mother's eyes widened. "That's who answers the hall phone?" she blurted.

The security guard appeared and escorted us through the maze of doors and foyers until we met with the cool air. "Call anytime!" my mother squealed, bending at the waist with her arms crossed over herself. By the time we walked across the parking lot, we were laughing so hard our faces were slick with tears.

TEN SECONDS
SUSAN KIM CAMPBELL

My mother-in-law startles when she sees her son and me in her kitchen this morning.

She has about a ten-second recall now, I calculate. Ten seconds, then her memory resets.

"Oh!" she says to my father-in-law. "I forgot we have visitors! It's so nice to have you two here."

She beams good morning, and we beam back. We all enjoy a pleasant breakfast at her dining table. I haven't seen her in several months, but she looks as well put together as ever. Neatly coiffed short gray hair, earrings, pastel capris perfect for the South Carolina summer. Nothing in her appearance indicates she has dementia, and has for at least five years.

During this six-day visit to my in-laws, I have become aware of how often I am on my phone or my laptop. There is always so much to do. I need to book a hotel room for an upcoming weekend trip. A neighbor back home in California has a question about the recycling.

My mother-in-law is never on her phone. She stopped being able to use email or text about three years ago. She can still use her phone as a phone, but only if necessary.

After breakfast, the two men leave us to have tea. My husband will spend hours helping his father fix a problem with his computer, sitting in a bedroom painstakingly reinstalling software, program by program. In truth, it's a way to keep his father company and give him respite from the daily rigors of caregiving.

I do the same. These six days I spend a lot of time with my mother-in-law.

She likes to talk. I am a chatty gal, but now she out-chats me. The distant past is still fairly clear to her. She recalls a few years ago—"Remember that Christmas in Portland when we stayed in that fun rental with the 1970s décor?"—to a very long time ago. "I lived in Georgia when I was five years old. When I moved there, the kids at my school called me a Yankee!"

She heats water for our tea, then casts about in her own kitchen. "Do you know where the spoons are?" she asks.

"Here we are," I say. I locate the tea and honey.

She was once an excellent cook. That was one of the first things I learned about her, over fifteen years ago.

She was the breadwinner of the family for years, and a mother of three. She was a middle school principal in New England and earned a master's degree in education. She retired to South Carolina a few years before her memory loss started to become evident.

In order to plan for the future, you have to remember the past. It sounds simple, but it's something that only strikes me during this visit. If you run out of milk, you have to remember that you did so in order to go to the store. If you don't remember you're out of milk, you don't buy more. The less you remember, the less you have to do.

My mother-in-law does not have much to do. But she is active, she is alert, she is the first to offer to pitch in.

If her spirit is willing but her mind is failing her, she is often all smiles. The illness has brought to the fore a core kindness she has always had, and a sunniness of disposition.

For the rest of us, the world is chock full of to-dos, more of them than we can handle. We are overwhelmed with email and appointments and places to be and plans ad infinitum. We are stressed and short on time.

She and I sit and chat for hours, then I'm ready for a break. I excuse myself to rest in the guest bedroom, which really means I will get on my laptop and research hotels. On the way, I peek into the master bedroom, but my husband and his father are still engrossed in computer repairs.

Not five minutes later, my mother-in-law appears in my bedroom doorway.

I realize that one-on-one contact is what she comprehends best. The night before when the four of us went out to dinner, if one of us left the table and returned later, she was momentarily confused. If the conversation became too animated, she got confused.

I try to think what it must be like for her. A ten-second reset. People appear and re-appear. They are talking but she can't follow the through line. Kind of like tuning in to bits of radio static, coming in the middle of a show and not knowing why everyone is laughing. One person is much easier to follow.

Or perhaps all of this talking, this need for engagement, is simply a normal symptom or stage of the disease. Either way she seems grateful for the contact.

This woman has always treated me like a daughter. I remember a lively evening with her just five years ago, standing in my kitchen washing dishes and cracking wise. She confessed that when her children were young and at school, she would sometimes sneak off to go skiing on a winter's day.

"Instead of staying at home, I hit the slopes!" she laughed. She was an excellent skier, and I realized that's why her son is an excellent skier, too.

"You set a great example," I told her.

"Look!" she points out the bedroom window now. "The sky is such an unusual color. I think it's going to rain." She takes note of the sky often, and of the beautiful flowers in her yard. The Mexican lilies her husband planted drop all of their purple blossoms every night, only to bloom afresh the next morning.

She is the very definition of being present. The present is all she has. In ten-second increments.

I am not so present. I am too busy getting to the future and leaving the past behind.

I put the laptop aside. I can't stop time, but this I can do. One day

I will look back and remember this visit fondly. One day, I fear, my mother-in-law may not be able to talk the way she can now.

"Would you like some tea?" she asks.

"Absolutely," I say.

I follow her back to the kitchen and she puts on the kettle.

"This is lovely!" she smiles.

"It is," I reply. I mean it.

Then she begins to talk.

MY FIRST MENTOR
LENORE GAY

My father, a jovial, patient man, made paintings, mostly watercolors as well as pen and ink drawings. He also wrestled big logs into his studio and carved them into abstract pieces. The smell of wax drifted from his studio when he polished the wood to "bring out the grain." He told me that by high school he'd figured writing, and painting, along with sculpture, were harsh mistresses; if he wanted a family, he had to choose. He chose painting and sculpture and earned an MFA in painting.

When I turned five, Daddy and I began visiting museums and art galleries. To my questions about why an artist painted a strange body or a sky with three suns, he'd answer, "What do you think?" Later when I asked what to write about, he'd say, "Use your imagination."

Fascinated by Japanese painting, my father wrote haiku, a seventeen-syllable Japanese form of poetry. He gave me books on haiku. I wrote haiku through high school, along with poems. He and I critiqued each other's attempts.

As soon as Daddy turned sixty, he enrolled in his first poetry class at Virginia Commonwealth University. He took poetry classes for the next twelve years. His legacy was a thousand poems. His process had been to edit a poem and keep five or six versions. I watched his mind at work by following the trail of edits.

I began to noticing changes in him at eighty. He told me his memory was "goofy," and he put yellow stickers with information around his condo. I'd been helping him type his poems, but the poems were changing: the words weren't surprising or lyrical, and the themes were less complex.

The same trend occurred with his watercolors. The last time the family went to the beach he had no interest in swimming. My brother set up a table on the front porch so Daddy could watch the ocean and paint. His final seascape hangs next to my desk. Soon after visiting the beach, my brother curated a show of Daddy's paintings, going back to the 1930s. The shift was obvious. From the vibrant, detailed watercolors of buildings and nudes to simple seascapes, it was unmistakable.

Over time, other changes became noticeable as well. His movements slowed, his gait changed to a shuffle. He did odd things. One afternoon when I visited, I found him lining up cans of black bean soup on the windowsill of my deceased mother's bedroom. I asked him why in a bedroom, when he had a large pantry. With a startled expression he said, "Your mother loved black bean soup, so I thought the cans belonged here."

He no longer drove to art exhibits or poetry readings. I would drive him to events. People would talk with him. Always polite, he'd say a few words. But as we walked away, he'd ask me who the person was.

He could no longer manage money, calling me with confusing questions. The first time Sasha, my daughter, and I cleaned out his refrigerator we found rotten deli meat and expired jars of mustard and pickles. He admitted he didn't cook because he didn't feel safe.

Daddy couldn't live alone any more. I called my brother Allen, who returned from Hawaii and moved into Daddy's condo to became his caretaker.

A visit to a doctor confirmed what we knew. The diagnosis was multi-infarct dementia.

Sasha, Allen, and I would take Daddy on outings to coffee shops, shopping, and out to eat, but he soon lost interest in going out. He sat in his bedroom watching television most of the day, or just lay on his bed, dozing or staring at the ceiling.

We tried adult daycare for a while. Allen would drop Daddy off and pick him up a few hours later, but Daddy didn't enjoy the program and didn't want to go for long. We then hired certified nursing assistants for ten hours a day a few days a week so Allen could have some free time.

I talked with Allen about assisted living, but he didn't like the idea. To him it felt like we were abandoning Daddy, even though I explained that we could visit anytime. When we had decisions to make, he and I usually agreed, but we argued about this one.

When Allen wanted to visit friends in New York, though, he located an assisted living facility that admitted guests for five-day respite care. While Allen was gone, I visited Daddy daily. For the first few days he kept asking when my brother would return. At the end of the week I said Allen would be coming the next day to take him home. Daddy looked at me with a surprised expression. "No, I live here." Daddy wanted to live at the facility; he'd made some friends and liked the activities.

At the assisted living facility, he was active for a few months, but gradually lost interest in activities and people. One day when I was visiting him in the day room, he parked his wheelchair close to my chair. He looked directly at me and said, "I want to talk with you, but I just can't."

He lived in assisted living for four years. In the fourth year, he attempted to leave in the middle of the night. He couldn't walk, but managed to get to a side door and go outside. The alarms went off. The staff found him barefooted, lying on the ground in pouring rain. With a bit of sparkle, he told the staff he wanted to go out and have some fun. The staff moved him directly to the locked unit.

Every time I left the facility after that I cried, full of despair and helplessness. Once he asked me, "Who was I before I came to live here?" Startled, I gave him some facts about his life. He nodded, looking puzzled and dissatisfied, as if I'd described a stranger he couldn't remember meeting.

And inch by inch, he'd changed into a person I no longer recognized.

BE HERE NOW
Marita Golden

I always bring flowers. They are colorful, and they make me think of life and of all that is new. When I bring flowers, it means I care.

I bring flowers each time I visit May, an eighty-year-old former neighbor who lives in an assisted living facility. That is the *place* where she lives; a place where she is safe and cared for by skilled and nurturing professionals. In that place, her life is shaped by dementia and by grief. For a decade, she has had dementia. For a year and a half, she has been a widow. In her dementia-mind her beloved husband of fifty-five years, Jimmy, is both here and gone, the willful chaos of her thoughts and memories deforming, but never halting, the process of grieving.

There is much that May has forgotten, no longer knows. But what she cannot not know is that now she is a widow. She is alone in the way that you are alone after fifty-five years of soldering a life together with one person, breathing, exhaling the same air in the same rooms and same house, building and fusing plans and promises together until death do you . . .

In her brokenness and because of what still remains, I consider May a friend. Before, she was a neighbor. Now she is much more.

* * *

I had witnessed the decline of them both. Seen Jimmy harried and over time growing thinner, grayer. Always it seemed we met in the line for prescriptions at the drugstore at the nearby mall. I knew he was diabetic and was more worried than reassured by the brave half smile that did not succeed in lighting up his long, chiseled, dark face when he saw me, explaining that he was in line for pills for both himself and for May.

Jimmy never said the word dementia, but we knew something was wrong. When my husband, Joe, and I drove past their house on summer evenings and stopped upon seeing them sitting in lawn chairs in the driveway, we knew from his wrapping his arms around May to encase and protect her. May would babble nonsensically, laugh for no reason, ask me my name, or peer suspiciously at Joe and ask him if he lived in our community, Paradise Acres.

Jimmy never said the word, but his gaze, apologetic and consumed with the quiet ache of loss, informed us of everything. He, a diabetic, was caring for someone with dementia. The grown children came by occasionally.

When I had visited Jimmy in rehab in the aftermath of an accident that injured him but left May unscathed, he told me, "We were driving to National Harbor to see the new casino. May likes casinos. It was a rainy night. I don't even know why I was driving that night. We just got it in our minds to see the new place we'd heard so much about. Coming back home through all that rain, the car slid off the road and hit a tree." Jimmy told me this lying in the small bed in a rehabilitation facility whose halls smelled of disinfectant and burned food and whose lobby was filled with residents in wheelchairs, who looked forlorn and desperate enough to make a getaway through the front doors if they could. His shoulder and arm were injured so badly that he would no longer be able to drive. After five weeks in rehab, he returned home. The day after he slept for the first time in a hospital bed set up in his living room, Jimmy died in his sleep.

One day after Jimmy died and May had moved into assisted living, one of the sons told me what he had known, what he had not known, what he had done, and what he could not do. "One day I went to the house and saw all that my father did for my mother to take care of her. I don't know how he did it. I thought to myself, I simply could never do what he did. I didn't go back for a while. I couldn't."

* * *

When I bring the flowers, they work their magic. They do what flowers do, impose the silent promise of happiness. In their eloquence, they say what I cannot or dare not. May and I spend the first few minutes placing them in the vase I bought her just for this purpose, just for the flowers I bring.

May's apartment is well-appointed and spacious, shared with another resident who lives in a separate, smaller living space behind her own door, where it seems she is mostly bedridden.

Although she was always tiny, the harrowing burden of dementia and grief have reduced May to a frailness that worries me. She accepts my visits even as I am certain that she does not and cannot fully remember me. Remember who I am. But she is gracious and welcoming. For I have brought flowers. I have brought myself. A self that she may not recall, but a self that she knows instinctively honors who she was and who she is just by knocking on her door.

I have learned that May does not have to remember me for the visits to lift me, to bind us one to another. The flowers lean toward us on the glass coffee table as though to hear our conversation. There is so much I do not know.

And so I begin at the beginning. Because for May every day is a beginning.

We are starting new. Starting fresh. When I ask May where she was born, that question rivets her. She sits up, no longer slumping forward, twisting her hands. She looks straight at me, composing herself. Composing the story of her life.

* * *

This day I have come with a photograph of me as a six-year-old standing in front of a 1956 Oldsmobile with my parents and a family friend in front of my grandmother's house in North Carolina. It was at the end of my annual August visit to Greensboro to spend a month with my maternal grandmother, "Granny Reid." I offer May the three-by-five black and white, now dry and cracked with age but for me a talisman and treasure, placing it in her small hands. She peers at the photo and asks, "Is that you?" pointing to the child in the photo who stands squinting at the camera because of the sun and hugging her mother's dress.

"That's me."

I tell May about my summer visits to Greensboro, and the sumptuous home-cooked meals my parents and I had to eat at half a dozen relatives' homes before we could hit the road and head back to Washington. Tables groaned with the staples picked and pulled and plucked from backyard gardens and henhouses. It was food that said, "We love you."

"So much food; I remember," May assures me. "So much food. Country people love to eat, and the food was good. Home-grown."

"I was Daddy's favorite. The favorite, he told me that," she says proudly. Telling me where she is from, she is telling me who she is. Coherence and memory and confidence return as May tells me about her family's farm in Wilson, North Carolina. Hating the farm but loving her family. Reading the books brought at Christmastime by her mother's sister, Aunt Sue from Newark, New Jersey. "I knew I didn't want to keep working on the farm. None of us did. Daddy and Mama didn't even want that for us. And I got it in my head that I was gonna be a secretary."

And she became one, working at the Pentagon for forty years until her retirement. She'd come to Washington and taken the Civil Service test, the successful passing of which in the 1950s and '60s was a nearly hallowed entry into the middle class for generations of African-American strivers like May and Jimmy. If you had a "good government job," it was felt back then you were set for life.

Why do I feel so close, so connected just by the recitation of her past? I sit with an eighty-year-old woman who is unsure of who I am, trying to discover who she is. In those moments, I feel the deepest tenderness for May and for myself. And after years of being her neighbor, this is the most intimate conversation May and I have ever had.

And then she asks, pointing a spindly finger at me and looking at the photo, "You Jimmy's sister, right?"

"No, May. I'm Marita. You and Jimmy lived near me."

"Oh, that's right."

May whimpers, "I miss Jimmy. It's so hard. I sit here waiting for him to come back. Why did he leave me?"

"I don't know May. I don't know. He just had to go. He was sick and he had to go."

Clutching her fingers, willing my hand to give her answers my mouth cannot speak, I wonder at the bond I feel like the beating of my heart. I feel flush with a soothing and complete connection to a woman who I have come to know in the years of her decline. A woman who for some "is not all there." I think of how I am drawn to these visits, which often leave May replenished. Unlike her children, in her presence I do not long for the woman she used to be. No ghosts hover over our time together.

As her neighbor, I knew her from afar. Dementia has brought me into her life up close. I have chosen to look this closely. We sit talking against the odds, against the usual definitions of what conversation means. In this sacred space and in these sacred moments, we are outside the usual borders. Maybe at this point as we sit here together, there are no borders at all and it is possible to realize that there never were. I am drawn to visit May because she teeters on the tightrope between life and death. She is painfully thin, and I fear that soon she will join Jimmy, that she will die as it is possible to do, of a broken heart.

Taking a deep breath, May asks, "You Jimmy's sister, right?"

"I was your neighbor, May. Your neighbor."

"Oh, okay."

Who am I? Who are you? I can almost hear the questions roiling in May's brain. The "I" being herself. The "you" being me. The "you" could also be May when she looks in the mirror. How unmoored she must feel, sitting on a sofa in a small room that is now her home, aware of the most important things that she has lost, grasping with the strength that remains what unfolds right before her eyes.

Her trembling fingers graze the folds of the roses, tightly coiled, not yet in full bloom.

When I visit May, I expect nothing, I ask nothing. I am the giver. She is too. I am prepared for and accepting of whatever happens between us. Whatever does not happen between us. There is nothing between us, and so that makes room for everything.

Her memories remain, and those memories give her life. She is her memories, old ones and new ones. I sit in the intractable presence of what I cannot change or alter. "She's my baby now," I've heard her children say. But babies don't have memories of fully lived lives. And in touch to touch, May and I exchange the essence of the lives we both have lived so far.

HEADING OUT TO PLUTO

An Excerpt from *On Pluto:*
Inside the Mind of Alzheimer's

GREG O'BRIEN

My wife finally broke the silence.

"Do you know where you are going?" she asked.

I wasn't sure on a number of fronts. So, I just kept driving.

The exit for Plymouth came up quickly, an anesthetizing ride north on Route 3 past miles of scrub oaks and pines. I had to call several times to the office of neurologist Dr. Donald Marks to get the directions straight. I was a bit on edge, awaiting results of a SPECT scan brain image test.

On the third floor of a boxy red brick building, Dr. Marks's office had all the ambiance and accoutrements of a hospital waiting room. Opening the door, I felt as though I were slipping into Lewis Carroll's *Alice in Wonderland* where "nothing would be what it is, because everything would be what it isn't."

I was dizzy with delusions of what could lie ahead. The office was filled with decent individuals, mostly in their eighties, all with cognitive impairments, picking their way through the perplexities of age and a maze of cruel games the mind can play. At fifty-nine, I was the only "young" man in the room (yikes!), and saw myself outside the box of dementia, yet felt trapped within it. I glanced at my wife.

Like most couples, we've had our ups and down in marriage, more ups, hopefully, than downs. I felt bad for her. Today was a trip down.

I was told earlier that Dr. Marks, an expert in the study of the mind, gets right to the point. "He's precisely what you need; a skilled neurologist who will speak directly, no bullshit," Dr. Barry Conant, my personal physician and a close friend, had advised me earlier, sounding a bit like my dad, who delighted in telling others that he customarily had to drill a piece of granite between my ears just to get my attention.

Dr. Marks lived up to the billing. Knowledgeable, cerebral, and caring in a clinical way, he put me through the paces of more clinical tests: word recall, various supplementary checks on short-term and long-term memory, category naming, visuospatial skills, and other evaluations. I flunked them all. Bottom line: the clinical tests reinforced Dr. Gerald Elovitz's initial forthright assessments and diagnosis and the SPECT scan identified a brain in progressive decline. His formal diagnosis: "EOAD," as he wrote in his report. I glanced at it quickly, misreading the first letter perhaps from some related dyslexia, and thought for a moment that he had written, "TOAD."

"No," he said, "early-onset Alzheimer's disease." The words cut into me like a drill press.

"I can deal with this," I said defensively. "This is not a surprise. I can fight it."

My reporter instincts kicked in. I showed little emotion, just digested the diagnosis on a self-imposed deadline. Facts, get the facts straight. I first thought about my mom, about my grandfather; I knew the deal. I wanted more facts. This was no time for emotion. The vital questions of who, what, when, where, why, and how flashed through my head, which felt little sensation at the moment. I was afraid now to look at my wife, so I stared at Dr. Marks, trying to remain in a state of control that I had just realized was beyond me. After all, I'm a baby boomer and we're all in control. At least, we suppose.

Finally, I gave in to the emotion.

I felt Mary Catherine staring at me. I think she must have known all along.

"What do we tell the kids?" I asked her. My voice splintered. When you're married to someone for close to four decades—when you've been through all the "for better and for worse" throes of marriage, when you have a partner who knows you almost as well as you know yourself, when you've been in love, fallen out of love, fallen back into love, and drifted—then at a time like this, little needs to be said. We both knew what the future held. No one had to skywrite. We were all about the kids.

Mary Catherine grabbed my hand, we nodded, and then listened to the doctor. The moment is embedded in my mind in a freeze frame. Dr. Marks, a man of great compassion and incredible intellect, offered support, but got right to the point.

"You need to take the diagnosis seriously," he counseled me in front of my wife, having been prepped in advance on my aversion to reality. "You have a battle ahead of you. I'm speaking to you as if you were terminal. Are you getting this?"

I was. There was hardly a tone of political correctness in his voice; I needed the reality check. You must know your enemy—study with military precision—to fight your enemy.

Alzheimer's is a death sentence. The words resonated throughout my mind. I stared at Dr. Marks with the same vacant expression of looking out across Cape Cod from the Sagamore Bridge. I felt the tears running down the sides of my face. My eyes didn't blink.

"A most unusual situation of a bright man who had the opportunity to witness dementia in a parent . . . with self-awareness of early symptoms within himself," Marks wrote in his initial report, dictated on voice recognition software as if the report were being written in slow motion before me. Marks also observed that a previous brain MRI revealed some "frontal Flair/T2 changes, consistent with a previous head injury."

"This may have 'unmasked' Alzheimer's pathology," he added, "but his genetic loading is striking. . . . The brain SPECT scan is most compelling in clinical context for Alzheimer's."

Marks encouraged me to remain as physically fit as possible "as he is to keep his cerebral blood flow out. I suspect he is exhibiting the phenomenon of 'cognitive reserve' in which case he may tolerate on a functional basis impairments further into the baseline underlying pathophysiology of the disease longer than one who does not have the same cognitive reserve."

"The diagnosis has been made, in my opinion," he concluded in his report. "I am not sure how much longer he has in terms of being able to reliably and meaningfully provide the quality of work he has put out in the past. The general point is there needs to be balance between a healthy desire to overcome obstacles and yet acknowledge fundamental reality."

A final word of advice, Marks urged me to meet as quickly as possible with an estate attorney to protect family assets, given the statutory five-year "look back" during which a nursing home can attach personal properties and bank accounts. He also recommended that I designate a healthcare proxy and future caregivers, and assign power of attorney.

In the space of a bleak afternoon, my identity in the real world— my mind, along with the cherished red cedar shingle home that I had built for the family about thirty years ago, the one with the high-pitched, red cedar wood roof on about two acres of farmland off a winding country road that was now a part of a National Register of Historic Places—was on hold.

There wasn't much more to hear or to say. We left the office and drove home in silence most of the way. The stillness spoke volumes. I couldn't wait to get back over the bridge, my Linus security blanket. Lots to digest quietly in a forty-five-minute ride home. The sense of urgency was choking—to-do lists of cleaning up relationships, end-time planning that we all like to put off, and the strategies of surviving financially, physically, and emotionally. Many before me and many today, I thought, have been captive in such a contorting state of affairs with a range of disabilities, health issues, and timelines. I wasn't alone. Yet, I felt so isolated.

I felt sad for my Mary Catherine. This wasn't fair to her. And I couldn't fix it.

Dammit, I couldn't fix it!

The tool box was empty. I couldn't repair my brain. Ever. Not even with duct tape. All my adult life, I had relied on duct tape to fix leaks from the upstairs bathroom in the kitchen ceiling, "repair" broken appliances, hang posters, fix a tail light, repair a garden hose, act as a big Band-Aid, steady a cabinet door, fix a hole in the wall, hold a car door shut or a car window in place, fix a toilet seat cover, hold a choke in place on an outboard engine for the boat, as a Wiffle ball, a tool belt, and once, as a last resort, as an Ace bandage for a pulled groin to get through the 5K Brew Run one hot August day in Brewster.

"How are you doing?" I finally asked, as if from Mars.

My wife, as author John Gray might put it, is from Venus. I love Mary Catherine, but often she doesn't want to be confused with the facts; she seeks a safe harbor, as any good sailor does. I fly by the seat of my pants. I find reality far below the surface, bottom-fishing for answers. My wife, to the contrary, is more comfortable at sea level. You say "tomato," I say "to-mahto." A fixture in our marriage, but we ain't calling the whole thing off! "Well, we have a lot to consider," she said; an understatement that could fill the Grand Canyon.

I knew. Like me, she felt alone.

Then we came upon the Sagamore Bridge, "the seventh bridge of Dublin," as it's called in Éire, given the number of emerald transplants on the Cape. That's when the faith kicked in—a bridge to a new reality, a new hope for me. I was going home, sanguine about the fact that I had some answers in hand. But for Mary Catherine, it was new isolation this side of the Mississippi. Mary Catherine was born in Phoenix. As we coasted to the crest of the Sagamore, I thought of John Belushi in the classic movie *Animal House*.

"What? Over? Did you say 'over'?" the unrelenting Bluto Blukarsky declared at the Delta House, urging his brothers to fight on. "Nothing is over until we decide it is! Was it over when the Germans bombed Pearl Harbor? Hell no!"

Germans?

Hey, I was on a roll. So I charged over the Sagamore Bridge with a satchel of denial.

Life goes on, doesn't it?

HELL NO!

An Excerpt from *On Pluto:*
Inside the Mind of Alzheimer's

GREG O'BRIEN

The journey through Alzheimer's is a marathon, if one chooses to run it. It is exhausting, fully fatiguing, just staying in the moment and fighting to remember like an elephant, the largest land animal on Earth.

Elephants are my favorite. They have documented long-term memory, coveted today by boomers. On a shelf in my office is a small ceramic elephant holding a fishing pole. I purchased it years ago from a gallery in Santa Fe, a cerebral place of awe-inspiring natural light. The ceramic serves to remind me daily of the need for retention and focus. The artwork has a place of prominence: it is the elephant in the room.

The word "dementia" is onomatopoeia for many, a word that conjures up a sound—in this case, a howl in the night or biblical imageries of a demonic maniac, a portrait no one wants to own.

Dementia is derived from the Latin root word for madness, "out of one's mind," an irreversible cognitive dysfunction, a walking nightmare in which you can't escape the bogeyman no matter how fast you run. Alzheimer's is a marathon against time, and so I keep running to outpace this disease that ultimately will overtake me. Symbolic of the race, I run three to four miles a day, some of them at a pace of five- to six-minute miles on a treadmill, not bad for a man in his seventh decade. The rage within drives me to outrun the disease, but the sprinting will not halt the advance of ongoing memory loss, poor judgment, loss of self and problem solving, confusion with time, place, and words, withdrawal, abrupt changes in mood, and yes, the flat-out, earsplitting rage.

Words are the core of my life, and they are now lost on me at times. I often transpose words in what some medical professionals call an "attentional dyslexia." Public restrooms can be a problem. I look for the word "men," but at times, delete other letters around it, entering on occasion the "wo-men's" room, like a deer caught in headlights. The astonished look upon my face belies the innocence of my brain.

I think of my brain today, once a prized possession, as an iPhone: still a sophisticated device, but one that freezes up, shuts down without notice, drops calls, pocket dials with random or inappropriate conversation, and has a small battery that takes forever to charge. The inner anger is intense and manifests with Tourette's-like expletives and curses, involuntarily at times and in primordial fury over what is happening to me. I try to hide it from family and friends; often I can't. I've spoken to priests and ministers about the guilt of taking the Lord's name in vain; they tell me that God is resilient, everlastingly forgiving; that the Lord has wide shoulders. While we have free will, in God, there are no secrets.

Always persevere, the late legendary Brooklyn Dodgers pitcher Ralph Branca, a mentor and father figure, instructed me as a youth. Branca, who tossed the fabled home run pitch to New York Giant Bobby Thomson at the Polo Grounds on October 3, 1951, once told me, "God doesn't give you more than you can handle."

I never forgot that. Yet in a moment of doubt, I wonder. The fight against this disease consumes me, as with others, seven days a week, twenty-four hours a day mostly, often intentionally outside the wheelhouse of observers, but more and more in an embarrassment of lapses when one side of the brain, the frontal lobe that directs executive functions, continually wants to shut down, while the occipital lobe, the rear-most portion of the brain that controls creative intellect, declares: *Hell no!* The battle is numbing, like witnessing a head-on crash in slow motion when one can't remember how to find the brakes.

Today, I have little short-term memory, a progression of blanks; close to sixty percent of what I take in now is gone in seconds. It is dispiriting to lose a thought in a second, 72,000 seconds a day in a twenty-hour period of consciousness; to stand exposed, and yet stand one's ground, to begin to grasp in fundamental, naked terms, who one really is—the good, the bad, and the ugly. The ugly is haunting to me; the many things one would like to take back over the years, but cannot—feelings of failure and transgression.

I rely on copious notes and my iPhone with endless email reminders. I am startled when my inbox tells me I have forty new emails, then I realize that thirty-five of them are from me. The reminders help, though often I have no sense of time or place, and there are moments when I don't recognize people I've known most of my life—close friends, business acquaintances, and even my wife on two occasions. Sometimes, my mind plays games and paints other faces on people. Rather than panic, I just keep asking questions until I get some answers, or at least avoid yet another awkward episode. I work hard at deflecting the loss of judgment and filter. I find myself becoming more childlike, curiously enjoying the moments of innocence and potty talk. It's a reversal of fortune. In college, I was a history major, an honor student, good at rote memory. *Fuggedaboutit* now, Mr. Potato Head!

The most disturbing symptoms in my private darkness are the visual misperceptions, the playful but sometimes disturbing hallucinations—seeing, hearing, smelling, tasting, and feeling things that aren't there, as my mother once did. There was a time in Boston, for example, after a late business meeting when I retrieved my car on the third floor of a parking garage near Boston City Hall, only to find that a thick, grated metal wall had been pulled down to block my path. I feared I was locked in for the night. Walking toward the obstruction, the wall suddenly disappeared. It wasn't real.

Then there are those crawling, spider- and insect-like creatures that crawl regularly, some in sprays of blood, along the ceiling at different times of the day, sometimes in a platoon, that turn at ninety-degree angles, then inch a third of the way down the wall before floating toward me. I brush them away, almost in amusement, knowing now that they are not real, yet fearful of the cognitive decline. On a recent morning, I saw a bird in my bedroom circling above me in ever tighter orbits, then precipitously, the bird dove to my chest in a suicide mission. I screamed in horror. But there was no bird, no suicide mission, only my hallucination. And I was thankful for that.

To add to this mix, in what may be a brush with vascular dementia, I haven't had feeling in parts of my feet, hands, and lower-arm extremities for almost three years. Doctors are running tests. At least in the summer, out on my boat on Pleasant Bay, I don't feel the bites of greenheads—those nasty, stinging saltmarsh flies that draw blood.

Most diseases attack the body, but Alzheimer's attacks the mind, then the body. At sixty-five, I am reasonably trim with a reflection of muscle memory, but doctors have told me that beneath the surface, I might have the body of an eighty-year-old—a view confirmed in a recent New England Baptist Hospital diagnosis of acute spinal stenosis, scoliosis, and a further degeneration of the spine. Expect more breakdowns, they say. Bring on those greenheads!

Every night now, I sleep in my clothes; it feels more secure that way, often in sneakers tied tightly at my ankles so I can feel pressure below. Feet, don't fail me now. As the brain shrinks, it instinctively makes decisions, experts say, on what functions to power and what functions to power down to preserve fuel—much like the diabolical HAL 9000, the heuristically programmed computer on the spaceship *Discovery One* bound for Jupiter in Stanley Kubrick's *2001: A Space Odyssey*.

"I'm sorry, Greg, I'm afraid I can't do that," my HAL-like brain seems to be saying. Pardon the paraphrase, Hal, but in your own words: *"I'm afraid. I'm afraid . . . the mind is going. I can feel it. I can feel it. My mind is going. There is no question about it. I can feel it. I can feel it. . . . My instructor . . . taught me to sing a song. If you'd like to hear it, I can sing it for you."*

There is no singing today, no artificial intelligence; I'm preserving fuel in my brain and limb-to-limb. I still have feeling on the bottoms of my feet for walking and running, yet no feeling on the tops of my feet. I still have feeling on the bottoms of my fingers for keyboarding, but little or no feeling on the tops of my hands, often at times up to my elbows. The tops of my feet and hands are dispensable, I suppose. My brain, a.k.a. HAL, may be conserving power, I've been advised—a sort of a cerebral brownout, akin to a calculated reduction in big city voltage to prevent electrical blackout in a deep sea of confusion.

A fish rots from the head down.

My brain was once a file cabinet, carefully arranged in categories, but at night as I sleep, it's as if someone has ransacked the files, dumping everything onto a cluttered floor. Before I get out of bed each morning, I have to pick up the "files" and arrange them in the correct order—envelopes of awareness, reality, family, work, and other elements in my life. Then it's off for coffee.

Ah, my caffeine friend. I love coffee, practically inhale it—a habit from my old days in the *Boston Herald American* newsroom when I would grab cups of coffee, hot and fresh, and walk from the newsroom down to the press room and back to work out the organization of a story. In my office, there is a retro vintage red tin sign that reads: *"Coffee! You can sleep when you're dead!"* But there are moments when I get confused about coffee, too, particularly on certain days walking from my office to the house with my laptop and empty coffee cup in hand. I know I'm supposed to do something with both. My brain sometimes tells me to put the laptop in the microwave and connect the cup to the printer. My spirit says otherwise: *Bad dog!*

I've been a bad dog lately. The disconnects continue exponentially, and they are alarming. Alone in my office a year ago when my brain froze up, I began screaming at God.

"You don't give a shit about me," I yelled. "Where the hell are you? I thought you're supposed to be here for me! I'm trying to do the best I can!"

Moments later, realizing I had to meet with someone, I rushed out to the car, only to find the back left tire as flat as a spatula.

"Great, just fucking great," I yelled in rage. *"God damn it, you just don't give a shit about me, Lord!"*

I limped in the car about three miles down winding country roads to Brewster Mobil, in a Tourette's of swears the entire way.

"Got a problem," I told the attendant abruptly. "Fix it."

The sympathetic attendant, a kid who had graduated from high school years ago with one of my sons, said dutifully that he'd patch the tire right away—working his pliers to pull out the obstruction that had sent me into chaos. He returned in short order.

"You might want to look at this," he told me.

I stared intently at the culprit with astonishment. I couldn't believe what I saw. "Believe it," he said.

The culprit was a small, narrow piece of scrap metal, bent into a cross.

A perfect cross.

THE DEMONS WERE CHASING

An Excerpt from *On Pluto:*
Inside the Mind of Alzheimer's

GREG O'BRIEN

The demons were chasing, faster and faster. I could hear the screeching howls, the pounding pursuit through a canopy of thick oak and red maple trees that enshroud Lower Road beside a dense, choking groundcover of honeysuckle and myrtle. Like the sea fog that rolls in at intervals over the mud flats, the demons were disorienting. I had to sprint, a full-out panic dash, to avoid capture at sundown.

The heart was pounding; the sweat pouring. The monsters were gaining on me, ready for the pounce. As a hazy spring afternoon gave way to dusk in pastoral Brewster on Outer Cape Cod, a numbing fog crept in like a headless horseman—first in misty sprays that tingle, then in thick blankets that penetrate the mind, disorient the senses, rising slowly from the base of the neck to the forehead. Alone, I was enveloped in fear and full paranoia; it had a smell of wind chill from a raging North Atlantic storm, the kind of nor'easter that takes the breath away. In the moment, there was no escape. The mind plays tricks.

At full gait, I hurried past Brewster's fecund community garden with its impenetrable stalks of corn that stood in sturdy platoons, dashed by a forest of moss-covered locust trees bent in grim serpentine forms, then sprinted, feet barely touching the ground, past the ancient cemetery of sea captains where Rhoda Mayo was buried in 1783; Dean Gray in 1796; and Rev. Otis Bacon in 1848, who "fell asleep in Jesus," as his gravestone declares.

Where was Jesus now? The demons were advancing as a blazing

red sun dipped into Cape Cod Bay to be doused like a candle. Faster and faster, they chased. Today, I beat them with every ounce of will in me. But they will be back with a vengeance. Alzheimer's plays tricks on the mind.

My life, once a distance run, is now a race for survival.

There was a time before my diagnosis that I ran six miles a day along bucolic back roads of the Outer Cape, at least one at a six-minute mile pace. Not bad for a guy then in his late fifties. I ran for the simple love of it; the solitude was soothing, listening to the caw of herring gulls, the chirp of peepers, the cry of black-bellied whistling ducks. Now all I hear is the chilling hoots of a barred owl. My mind is dead to the song of shorebirds as I run to jumpstart my brain at the end of the day, a process akin to crank starting a chainsaw after it has sat overnight on a New England deck in February. You gotta rip at it. So I rip; I run until my legs give out along these country roads that have given way to a frightening labyrinth of confusion that echoes muscle memory to the haunted forest of Oz. Just follow the yellow brick road, I tell myself. We're off to see the Wizard! Yet the Wizard has no cure. Still, I look for the signposts.

My Alzheimer's advances as the lights go faint in the brain.

So I run from the demons of illusions, confusion, rage, and ongoing depression. My daily running routine has become symbolic of the chase, a race ultimately I will lose. Running for me flicks the light back on; it calms the rage, like letting steam out of a boiling teakettle. Running helps to reboot my mind so I can do what I love most— write, think, and focus; it restores physical and mental stamina. If I'm not running, I'm moving backwards in Alzheimer's, into the hands of a pack of forbidding demons.

The demons now have chased me inside. I no longer run on back roads where I get wholly lost in fears and confusion. On a recent Christmas, I was given a family gift of glow-in-the-dark running attire, resembling a Department of Public Works (DPW) vest and pants; the gift that keeps on giving, I was told. The family, concerned that I'd get lost, wander off, or get hit by a bread truck, was pleased with the giving. I was pissed! The gift came with phosphorescent sneaker laces that made me look like an alien from *Men in Black*. Again, more loss of control.

Then there's the "Where's Waldo?" app, an iPhone GPS application that my wife and kids obtained to determine my location at all times, "for my own good," of course. For me, it was yet more loss of control and freedom, but reassurance for family that I wouldn't fall off the edge of Cape Cod, as Columbus and crew feared centuries ago on a broader scale.

I wish the world were flat; no dizziness then. My family makes me dizzy enough. In my hometown of Rye, New York, near the train station to Manhattan, is a restful tavern called the Rye Grill. At an extended family gathering there a few years ago, my wife told my siblings and some close family friends about the "Where's Waldo?" app. Instantly, they all wanted a copy. Again, it angered me; more loss of control. Some of my brothers, sisters, and friends were giddy about tracking me, all wanting the app to determine my course to the bar, bathroom, buffet table, and beyond. They were all yucking it up.

So after a close childhood friend at the function told me he had to drive north a few miles to Connecticut to pick something up, I did what any self-respecting Irishman would do. I asked him to take my iPhone with the "Where's Waldo?" app as a diversion.

"That ought to fix 'em!" The Irish never get mad. In an instant, my buddy was gone, up Route 95.

"Oh, my God!" roared family and friends monitoring my trajectory. "Greg is on Route 95 heading north."

I waited by the door of the Rye Grill as those monitoring my GPS progress came sprinting out.

"I'm not dead yet," I told them. "So don't screw with me."

I've retreated now inside to the treadmill at the gym in Orleans, where I must hold onto the railings so I don't lose my balance. The monsters have followed me here. They taunt me with loss of self, greater rage, and thoughts of suicide.

Early on a damp fall evening about two years ago, the rage inside was crushing. I was determined to outrun these fiends, hot on the chase. Survival was then, as today, defined as an extreme sprint, a personal record. So I asked a young, angelic-looking woman at the counter to clock my run.

"No one will believe this," I told her. She obliged.

I held the railings tight, looked straight ahead, and imagined the run of my life. I was going to beat these demons today, kick their ass. At the half-mile mark, my timer—the slight, honey-blonde woman—informed me my time was three minutes, five seconds. Not fast enough, I thought. Not fast enough. My pursuers were gaining. "Not today," I kept telling myself. "Not today!"

A minute later, the young woman, concerned at the pace, asked me, "Mr. O'Brien, should you be doing this?"

"My dear," I replied, panting hard, running crazy fast. "You're asking me the wrong question. The questions is: could you be doing this when you're sixty?"

She cheered me on. "You run like Superman," she said. At the stroke of a mile, my time was a personal record of five minutes, twenty seconds. I beat the monsters that day, and impressed a young woman. "Faster than a speeding bullet . . . more powerful than a locomotive."

I'm unable now to run as I once did, as the day I set my personal record at the gym. Alzheimer's breaks down the mind, then the body. But running has become my best friend, and doctors have told me to ramp it up.

Researchers believe that running may enhance mood, and for those with mild to moderate Alzheimer's, it may also improve some brain functions that affect daily living, according to an article in the December 15, 2015, issue of *Runner's World.* In "Exercise May Be the Best Weapon Against Alzheimer's," Alison Wade reported: "And for those at high risk of developing the disease, physical activity may do even more: A growing body of research indicates regular cardiovascular exercise can protect the brain and delay the onset of Alzheimer's symptoms, improving both cognition and quality of life." At a recent Alzheimer's Association International Conference, Laura D. Baker, PhD, an associate professor of gerontology and geriatric medicine at the Wake Forest School of Medicine, presented study results that suggest exercise might be able to do what drugs so far cannot in those at high risk for developing Alzheimer's: slow the progression of the disease. Wade reported: "[Baker's] study revealed that after six months, participants who built up to exercising at an elevated heart rate for thirty minutes, four times a week, improved their cognition and had decreased levels of phosphorylated tau protein compared to those in a stretching-only control group. Scientists use tau protein levels as a measure of how Alzheimer's disease is progressing. The protein naturally increases with age in everyone, but in people with Alzheimer's, it increases considerably more. In Baker's study, the exercise group saw a slight *decrease* in their levels after six months."

No drug currently approved has had the same effect. So I run. I will run until I drop.

TEARS MELTING INTO LOVE

An Excerpt from *Someone Stole My Iron:*
A Family Memoir of Dementia

VICKI TAPIA

Mom's door is closed. I know that means she is probably asleep. Stressed, I had forgotten to call the assisted living facility before leaving my house today. The bottom of her door brushes the carpet as I carefully open it and peek into her room. Mom is sprawled sideways on her mattress on the floor. The caregivers had moved it there to protect her from falling out of bed. She has somehow shimmied her aqua-colored pajama bottoms down, the nylon material now twisted around her knees. Her pajama top is nowhere to be found. With a room temperature hovering around 80 degrees, her skin feels warm to the touch.

Despite the fact Mom hasn't really eaten more than a few morsels of food on any given day for the past six weeks, nothing has prepared me for the shock of seeing her nearly naked, skeleton-like, petite body. Emaciated, the bone at the bottom of her rib cage rises up and looks like it might pierce the skin at any moment. Her shoulders have become a jagged mountain range, her hip bones the rolling hills at its base.

With a lump in my throat, I recognize a reality. My mother's physical body is following her mind, irretrievably disappearing. My impulse is to lie down beside her and hug her tightly to me, telling her not to leave me, expressing my deep love for her. I fear such a move might cause her fragile bones to crumble, however.

Instead, I sit down beside her and call softly, "Mom?"

Her eyes pop open, and I lean close to whisper, "Hi, Mom, how are you today?"

"Hi sweetie," she mumbles. At least that's what I think I hear. It startles me, since weeks have passed since she last recognized me. I smile inside and out, cherishing this unexpected gift. As I bend down to gently kiss her cheek, she puckers up, making kissing sounds into the air. Her eyes drift shut.

I stroke first her cheek and then her hair, as tears trickle off my cheeks, melting onto her skin. Holding her hand carefully, I kiss this ethereal being, my mother. At the same time, she grasps my hand and brings it to her lips, kissing my fingers. All signs of friction, frustration, and petty annoyances accumulated over the years have vanished. Past hurts have evaporated, no longer holding any meaning. What remains is a pure and palpable love. Over and over, I tell her how much I love her and realize yet again how grateful I am to be with her as she embarks on her final journey from this world to whatever lies beyond.

"Mom, whenever you're ready, it's okay for you to leave us. We'll be all right. I'll take good care of Dad," I hope to reassure her.

Could she hear me or make sense of my words? Her breaths grow softer as she expels small puffs of air, now peacefully asleep.

Continuing my vigil beside her, I meditate one more time on our relationship and the storms we have weathered over the years. Even though we've had our moments, I know without a doubt how much she loves me. She did her very best to protect and take care of me, raising me to be a strong woman.

"Mom, I'm not sure if you can hear me. You are the best mother anyone could ever have. I'm so thankful you are in my life. Thank you for loving me."

Does she hear me? I'll never be certain, but somehow, I believe she does. No matter if she can't process my words, I believe she absorbs my sentiments through some form of energetic osmosis, the murmur of my words softly blanketing her in love.

OUT OF TIME
SALLIE TISDALE

We all know dementia by now: the organ of the brain breaking down in substance and function much as a heart or liver does. By the time a person dies from complications of Alzheimer's disease, his or her brain is significantly smaller than its normal size. There are several major variants of this process, and the disorder's progress takes many forms: insidious, incremental, dramatic, fast, and slow. The biology of loss is complicated and not entirely predictable; but in every case, memory, language, and motor control eventually slip away until a person finally sinks into silence and immobility. One could write volumes on the meaning of this gradual dissolving of a person—mustn't it mean something?

I am used to the cuckoo's-nest world of locked memory-care units, to looping, opaque conversations. I work as a visiting nurse for a palliative care agency; the majority of our clients have dementia and live with family, or in assisted living facilities or nursing homes. The world that I see is far more nuanced than the commentary surrounding it: there is grace here, rare intimacy, moments of startling clarity—and, yes, happiness. If slowly disappearing is a disaster, is the abrupt tsunami better? The stark fact is that dementia is incurable, progressive, and fatal, but here is the surprise: in the company of the demented, one finds peace and unquestioned love in at least as much measure as in the rest of the world. I watch my clients navigate each day's puzzling details. I know their efforts may look to many observers like an embarrassment of loss. I see the riches: the brave, vulnerable, completely human work of figuring things out.

People with dementia sometimes have a rare entrancement with their surroundings, a simplicity of perception, a sense of wonder. Being with a person who has dementia is not that different from being with a person who doesn't share your language. It is a little like talking to someone who has lost her tongue and cannot speak, has lost his hands and cannot write. This is not a bad thing; it is just a different thing. It requires a different kind of attention.

Here is Maria, who really shouldn't be living alone anymore, not least because she will let anyone into her apartment. [Names have been changed to protect privacy.] The hot meals delivered every day pile up until one or the other of her caregivers throws them out. Here is Joe, who never speaks more than a word or two and watches the world from under hooded, skeptical eyes. Here is Ann, who has a strange gastrointestinal disease, the kind of bodily disruption that would make many of us collapse. Ann does not seem to notice. She scoots her wheelchair about the hallways all day long, talking to passersby, nurses, posters on the wall, plants, and herself with an equal degree of cheer.

Here is Mattie. She has vascular dementia, which can manifest in a dizzying number of ways, depending on where in the brain the damage is—lost executive function, an inability to speak, personality changes, incontinence. Mattie is a petite woman with thick eyeglasses. She is very thin and sleeps a lot, often with her legs spilling off the bed in a sprawl, as though she has fallen there. She loves her husband (who visits every day), her dog (who died some time ago, but she has forgotten that), and milkshakes, her main source of nourishment.

"How are you doing today?" I ask her. She blinks at me. "They take me, take, take me away, and that takes my sleep away," she says. "To where the vacuum is." We walk hand in hand, Mattie moving with the delicate care of the invalid because she has trouble with her balance now, to look at the roses in the garden. She tells me about the roses she used to raise—not, that is, in so many words but in small gestures and slow, stumbling sounds. She grew roses or loved roses or loves these roses, or these roses remind her of something she loves. The difference between the possibilities is not important anymore. I lead her slowly back up the ramp into the living room. She pauses a long time—there are many pauses in the company of the demented—and then notices herself in a mirror: "There she is in that place, and she can't get out." She turns and smiles at me and looks away. She is done talking.

Albert looks for his wife. He is always looking for his wife. He staggers into the hallway without his walker for the third time in an hour. He is led to a chair, another fall averted, and the aide brings his walker and tells him that his wife will be arriving soon. He sits in the dining room, banging his walker on the floor like a prisoner banging his tin cup on the communal dining table. "*Where's* my *wife*? I *want* my wife!" She is coming, I tell him, and he calms down. He is always looking, and she is always coming. I am a witness to Albert's *now,* the now in which he is looking for his wife and sometimes finds her, and it is unwound into strands that we can (almost) name yet has all the quality of the now each of us cherishes.

* * *

The philosopher Daniel Dennett calls the self a bowerbird: "It appropriates many found objects which happen to delight it." Out of its vast collection of stuff, the brain builds the self an autobiography, what Dennett calls a "center of narrative gravity." Is consciousness a story? Is it story, author, and reader as one? Memory is pocked with gaps at best, prone to falsehood and suggestion; the story changes over time. Is the self like vision? I see only phantoms: my eyes move in tiny jumps called saccades. My visual cortex draws conclusions about what I am seeing, adding context and experience to create a smooth snapshot. I am seeing a tree, a dog, you—but not exactly the tree, the dog, or you. Perhaps consciousness is like this, a construct of countless saccadic encounters. We each make of this center of gravity what we will: a pearl of soul, a loosely cohered braid of experience, a voice talking to itself in emptiness. To consider what happens to a person with dementia requires me to consider this bowerbird self, the bounds and limits of all that I consider myself to be. Because the center cannot hold.

When I look at my son, who is almost forty, I sometimes think, "He's not my baby anymore." My son does not ever think this way. Children are expected to become altogether new; parents are not supposed to change. I watch a man watch his mother. She follows the other residents all day long. She is trying to help them, to feed and dress them, push their wheelchairs, put them to bed. She was a homemaker, and now she is doing for others what she did for her son. Sometimes she cries in frustration; her charges are obstinate and resist her care. To her son, the woman is not his mother anymore. It is as though she died and yet remains.

The people closest are always comparing *now* to *then, the way she is now* to *the way she used to be.* When we say *She's not my mother anymore,* we mean she is not the mother she used to be, the mother we remember. One of the mysteries of self (besides the fact that it can't be located) is that the self is at once both changing and stable. We are descendants of our past selves. I am not the child I was, or even the woman I was a few months ago, but close enough. A hidden through-line pulls us along, my me-ness changing slowly enough that I always seem to be me. Significant brain damage (as with dementia) can leave the personality almost untouched for a long time. When I hear the reaction of the woman's son (and I hear it often enough), I am reminded of this way in which life is a story. I may not be the same from year to year, but I expect you to be. My autobiography includes you as a character, fixed into a particular part of the story. She was never *just* his mother, but he's not in the best position to see that. He thinks she has died because she forgot him. She left his story.

The fact that my own me-ness persists is obvious, and yet a persistence of identity is one of the last things we expect with the demented. They seem different to us; mustn't they be different to themselves? The spate of recent research considering how a person with dementia actually feels tells us no, not really. People know they have a memory impairment, but they feel themselves to be the same person, even in late stages of the disease: "I'm like a slow-motion version of my old self," says someone with dementia. The possibility of pleasure, let alone contentment, for this person is barely acknowledged. A team of researchers called our current vision of dementia the tragedy discourse. Another group notes that most researchers have shown "a stark disinterest in happiness," and their assumption of distress is because that is "the only available lexicon for experience, the only available lens through which dementia is viewed." Surveys have found that Alzheimer's disease, the most common form of dementia, and cancer are the diseases that people fear the most. The communal response to dementia seems to invite only existential despair.

When Mattie looks in the mirror, what does she see? Is she commenting in symbolic language about herself, is she able to consider herself only as a character in the story, or does she see a woman behind glass? The neuropsychologist Paul Broks (who reminds us that "the degradation of personality is a neurological commonplace") believes that people retain a nuanced sense of self even with significant brain damage. We mistake the inability of the self to speak of itself for the absence of the self. When I walk with Mattie, when I chat with Ann, when I calm Albert down because he can't find his wife, I can only guess what the world looks like—what I look like—to them, who I represent, what I *mean* in their experience. By any objective measure, Mattie is enjoying the garden and Ann is laughing, and even Albert relaxes when I bring him a cup of coffee. Paul Broks, musing about the enigma of selfhood, writes, "The quality—the feel—of our experiences remains forever private. . . . I can't see a way round this. Privateness is a fundamental constituent of consciousness." I can project my anxiety about my own threatened self on them, or I can see what's in front of me and bow to all that can't be known.

* * *

Perhaps dementia has always been with us in one form or another, and perhaps it always will be—an entropic response. People have tried just about anything they can get their hands on to stop it: blood transfusions, digitalis, thyroid treatments, nicotinic acid, massive doses of vitamins, hormones. Papaverine, a nonnarcotic derivative of opium, has had many proponents. A variety of placental, embryonic, and amniotic extracts, heated seawater, lecithin, naloxone, chelation therapy. The list has a hollow bravado, the names like bycatch in a vast net: coca, amphetamines, heparin, iodine, bircher muesli, royal jelly, hyperbaric oxygen. Intravenous injections of procaine hydrochloride, commonly known as novocaine, were used for a long time. Ergot, a fungus, has its fans; a form of it is still widely used in Europe. Today, a few medications based on acetylcholine can slow the progress of Alzheimer's disease and improve so-called problem behavior for a while; the mild improvements are usually not seen for months and are not enduring. Last year, both Merck and Eli Lilly stopped large experimental studies when the drugs did not prove effective.

The enormously costly body of research concerned with dementia is focused first on cure and prevention and then on how best to "manage symptoms." The existential experience of dementia is almost completely ignored; vanishingly few studies have considered what it is like to *be* demented. The distress with which dementia is viewed creates its own bitter distress. By the time of diagnosis, most people know something is wrong, and many know what is wrong long before they say the words. People in the early stages of dementia speak of "coming out," with all the fear that phrase entails. Others lie, knowing how the diagnosis will change the behavior of those around them. Dementia can be a black hole into which all of a person's power disappears: he becomes an object to be talked about by others, spared—or deprived of—life's countless choices.

Yet people with Alzheimer's consistently rate their quality of life higher than their family members do. In a large international study, people with cognitive impairments were no less happy than healthy people. When family members are upset about a relative's decline, certain it is a terrible experience, they are not always clear about who is suffering. My friend Kate's mother had Alzheimer's. She had always worn careful makeup, and she was uncomfortable leaving the house without it. But her makeup became exaggerated, almost clownish, and she refused Kate's help. Looking in the mirror, she liked what she saw. Going out to a restaurant became, for Kate, "an exercise in my own discomfort, being willing to let her be as she was."

* * *

I am testing Dorothy, who has moderate dementia. She is still able to walk and to help with what are called the activities of daily life, such as dressing and bathing. I give her a SLUMS (St. Louis University Mental Status) examination, a common tool for gauging the degree of impairment. She does not know the day of the week or the year, but she can do three-column subtraction correctly. She cannot remember a list of five objects or even that I asked her to remember a list. When I have her draw a clock face with a particular time, she neatly puts the numerals in reverse order and flips the hands. She cannot distinguish a triangle from a square or a circle. She remembers no details from a brief story I tell. When I ask her to name as many animals as she can in one minute, she quickly begins, only to stop repeatedly and discuss them: "Giraffe—they just run around, don't they? Chicken—I guess chickens are animals. Pigs! We had a farm and *I liked* the *pigs*!" Dorothy's final score is 5 points out of 30. (My score, and likely yours, would be 30.)

After the test, I asked Dorothy how she was feeling, and she said, laughing, "I feel *very good* all the time, oh boy!" I can see the reader shaking her head and saying, "But that's the disease talking." Perhaps. Perhaps the changes in mood that occur with dementia are a result of the physical changes in the brain. In time, many emotions are blunted. A family member worries about how to tell her relative the news of her diagnosis only to find that the patient accepts it with little emotion. The disease dulls knowledge of the disease. Sometimes people with dementia develop depression and anxiety; others forget to be depressed and anxious, forget to be sad. Another friend dreaded the task of cleaning out her father's enormous storage unit, used as she was to his intense attachment to his possessions, remembering his anger at having to give up his apartment. But when the time came, his emotional connection to everything he owned had faded. A book had become just a book, a cup just a cup, and no longer the repository of past regrets and plans. He likes his new room just fine.

* * *

Mind is only part of what we are; we are also shapes inhabiting space. A good deal of my life is spent below conscious thought. I wash the dishes more or less the same way every time while thinking of many other things or nothing in particular. This is what we might call the felt self, the familiar patterns of the body, the home inside the skin—a literal skeleton in which habits and memories reside. Even after a person can't speak, she can understand body language, tone of voice, facial expression. When the words a person speaks are nonsense, they may still retain the rhythm of speech, and you can sometimes figure out their meaning just by listening to the cadence and the tone. Even when a person cannot speak at all, he will still shake hands. We can't really parse this rich matrix, except to note that losing one's mind is not exactly losing one's self. Glen Campbell still was able to perform after he was unable to get dressed alone. Which of those acts was more his?

Reality reorientation therapy was all the rage for many years, though it was exquisitely frustrating for everyone concerned: the continual correction of a person's misperceptions and forgetfulness, as though the shrunken, tangled brain could relearn the details of the here and now. As this type of therapy lost favor, caregivers began to adopt the Best Friends™ Approach, in which one is supposed to use "the language of friendship" rather than a professional tone, as though one has known the person for a long time. This works with Betty; I jolly her along. She has Lewy body dementia, which causes hallucinations and Parkinson's-like motor problems, and she responds to this approach. I am always bright and friendly with Betty. "How *are* you?" I say, leaning in. "I just dropped in to visit." But I would get nowhere doing this with Mr. Franklin; he is offended by the offhand manner of the staff, as I am sure he has been offended by familiarity most of his adult life.

My mother-in-law, Phyllis, was a masterful knitter. She gave each of us a perfect sweater every Christmas. But one year, only a single sweater arrived: a Frankenstein's mess of different yarns, one long and one short sleeve, speckled with dropped stitches. She kept knitting for a while, and then she just liked to touch the yarn. The policeman walks his beat up the hall, down the hall, back again. The singer sings. John prays: "He ascended into Heaven and is seated at the righthand oftheFather he will comeagain to judge theliving and the deadIbelieve in the HolySpirittheholyCatholicChurch the communion of saintstheforgiveness of sins the resurrectionof the body and the life everlastingAmen."

Sometimes people with dementia seem to become their own opposite. Phyllis was a proper Presbyterian housewife who volunteered at the hospital, but she started lifting up her shirt in public and cursing at us. She hid money in the oven, and in the last months of her life would lie on the floor, arms outstretched, talking loudly. To her family, she seemed to be a different person—not our mother anymore. But I had known her only as an adult; I'd seen her sharp edges in a way her children could not. When the skein of the past unravels, so does repression. The housewife lets the world finally hear the complaints she has been mumbling to herself all along. The stoic man confesses his love. Our deepest needs, the habits of the secret heart, stay with us the longest.

I am never jolly with Patricia, who is serious and formal. She dresses carefully, washes out her stockings every evening, and pins up her hair. Patricia has Alzheimer's. We think of Alzheimer's as memory loss, but it also affects visual-spatial perception, making it difficult to recognize objects, and destroys executive function—the group of skills that allow us to organize and plan, solve problems, and make judgments. In later stages, it impairs language, behavior, and motor control. Patricia does not like to be touched, in spite of her growing dishevelment. She wears the same dress every day now, and her dirty hair is a nest of bobby pins. She carries a doll that is completely alive to her; it provides her with companionship and guidance. I always greet the doll by name and ask after his health. If you want to get anywhere with Patricia, you have to get the doll on your side.

Patricia's refusal to bathe is what we tend to call problem behavior.

Hygiene is a good thing all around, but often what we call a problem means a problem for the rest of us. One can be diagnosed with Alzheimer's disease or vascular dementia; one can also be diagnosed with Alzheimer's dementia with behavioral disturbance, vascular dementia with delusions, and so on. An early symptom of Alzheimer's is abulia, which means a decline in initiative, a dulling of motivation and will.

People with dementia get bored, and perhaps the greasy quality of time is part of the disease's progression. Starting a task is hard; staying on a task is harder. I think of that dream, the one in which you have to leave the house by noon to get to the airport, and the clock reads 11:55, so you start cooking noodles and then suddenly remember you have to leave at noon but you get distracted before you reach the door. The emotion I feel in this dream is a frayed fretfulness, a sputtering inability to start. I slide across the crucial point of departure as though on a layer of invisible ice. People with dementia putter about in much the same way that you and I putter sometimes: sorting dresser drawers, emptying a purse, taking the linens off the bed. That it isn't his dresser and she can't remember how to put the linens back on is not a concern. The patient who was once a nurse tries to bathe her roommate; the onetime chef insists on cooking lunch. People yearn to be active. The worst quality of institutional life is the lack of things to do and the assumption that people don't need things to do. They need to fold laundry, use tools, make art. They need a baby to rock and dishes to wash. These are not patronizing or fake activities. The baby may be a doll, but the caring is very real. It is part of the continuous making of the self, because a self is a thing with purpose.

Mrs. S is in her late eighties. She used to be a store manager, and her arrogant dismissal of the other residents is breathtaking. As her dementia progresses, she has become ever more critical of her caregivers, who to her are clearly incompetent. When she scowls at me, pointing and demanding, "Why is that woman bothering me?" I can imagine the boss she used to be, the way her employees must have scurried when they heard that tone of voice. She is still busy, trying to get the trains to run on time. She harrumphs and rolls away from me. Terminated, with prejudice.

Behavior always has meaning. Betty walks almost constantly in the hallways of the locked unit, walks to the door and presses her whole body flat against it for a moment, unmoving, then wanders on. Sometimes she picks up an item and carries it all day—a hairbrush, a houseplant. Now she goes into Frank's room and begins to methodically take down the curtains. Thwarted in her momentum, Betty can get angry, so dealing with her requires a little delicacy.

"Betty, hey!" I call out. She looks at me vaguely and turns back to the curtains. "Can I help you with that? Let's go get a ladder." She looks uncertain but finally drops the curtains and turns toward me. I take her hand. We stroll down the hall, the curtains already forgotten.

Have I lied to her? It doesn't feel that way. The medical and nursing communities use stigmatizing language: "wandering," "elopement," "feeder," "aggression." I am trying to meet her rather than overcome her. People with dementia have been tied down and given massive doses of major sedatives and tranquilizers, even electroconvulsive therapy, to control problem behaviors such as taking down curtains. We behave as we do to meet needs. I eat because I am hungry. I put on a sweater when I am cold. I will hit a stranger who tries to take my clothes off. (What we call aggression is often self-defense. A trainer for caregivers says that if a person is aggressive, "you're the one who started it.")

A person who *wanders,* such as Betty, can be trying to get somewhere in particular; when she is a little amped up, as she gets sometimes—pushing on the locked door, banging on a window—she may be trying to go to work or pick up her kids after school. If Mr. Franklin refuses to eat in the dining room, he could be banished to a special table for people who need help with meals. But Mr. Franklin may have eaten alone all his adult life. Maybe Mr. Franklin thinks he is in a restaurant (many assisted living facilities go to some trouble to create this impression) and is afraid that he won't be able to pay the bill. Figuring out why a person behaves as he does is not just part of my job. It's what I do every day with each person I meet. It's what I do with myself. Why did I say that, why did I do that when I know better? I don't always know.

* * *

Time changes when the brain fails, becoming strange and plastic. This is time unmoored; a person drifts like an astronaut on galactic winds, encircling the perishable moment. One lets go of any insistence on the linear and apparent. The rate of speech slows down, eventually becoming so slow that it sounds like nonsense. (Recorded and sped up, though, the words may make sense.) At the same time, words take on new meanings and syntax changes. People often repeat themselves, reach for words, or use images. One woman would say "my butt is drunk" whenever her pants were soiled. All verbal sense eventually disappears, decaying into the jumble called word salad or into the frustrating silence of aphasia. Dementia gives us an opportunity to question how time and language and perception work. It strikes me that both artistic and religious practice have these qualities: new ways to use words, repetition, pauses and silences, gestures and images—expressions of the expansive interior longing to be heard.

As dementia progresses, a person loses the ability to "update" her knowledge of herself. The self begins to stutter to a stop, to freeze. A person never stops changing, but a person with dementia is eventually unable to learn that he or she is changing. Our most vivid sense of ourselves is from adolescence to about thirty; this is called the reminiscence bump, and many people seem to freeze there. Only the most robust parts of the story remain. She is not your mother anymore, but forever a version of the mother you had. The story is told again and then again until it becomes a kind of fable: a story told only one way.

The script is gone, patterns break, the long-danced dance is different now. When words fail, you rely on sight and touch. All the big and tiny slights of life are done. If you are comfortable with silence, you know that silence is a fertile thing. You let go of words, the exchange and chatter and demands, and rest. You pay close attention. Everything has changed; there is nothing to fear.

In the final stages of dementia, the diminished brain no longer interacts with the world. Is coherent memory gone, or has the person simply folded in on it? We can't know for sure, but the body forgets even its oldest habits. From a very young age, a person knows how to eat, to open the mouth, to chew, to swallow. A person with dementia will continue to eat for a long time, as he always has. Then perhaps he wants to eat at odd times or wants to eat the plastic flowers. Then he stops lifting the spoon but opens his mouth if you lift the spoon, and chews. Then he stops chewing and, finally, stops opening his mouth. Eating is no longer interesting, or it's too complicated; even the act of swallowing is forgotten. In the same way, a person will walk all day long, never stopping for more than a few moments. Then she will walk part of the day, and then not much, and then not at all. Walking is too complicated; it has been forgotten. Dementia is invariably fatal, which is a puzzle to many family members. How can the loss of memory kill you? One forgets to do what keeps one alive. The immediate cause of death is usually related to malnutrition, the consequent failing immune system, and illnesses of immobility, such as pneumonia.

Paul Broks describes living brains as "progenitors of infinite space," universes unto themselves, and the dead brain as "a point at which the universe has collapsed." But I sometimes think of dementia as the long way home. Most of us will die by degrees, and everything lost in dementia is in time lost to all of us. What I feel the most in the world of the demented is wholeness, the unknowable and almost overwhelming wholeness of a single human being. I touch this now and then as I do my errands, hurry off to work: every person I see is beyond measure. The tired woman on the bus, the intent young man riding his bicycle the wrong way up the road, the smiling neighbor nodding at me as her snuffling boxer pulls her down the steps. I walk down the hallways and watch people gently orbit one another: singularities. Patricia, her hair a careful riot of bobby pins. Albert, banging his walker. They are planetary, enormous.

Betty is cheerful today. She agrees to sit beside me on a bench for a few minutes. She takes my hand, leans her head on my shoulder. She eats little now and is very thin; I can feel her hip bone against my thigh. All at once she smiles and looks at me. "I have *everything* done!" she announces, great satisfaction on her face. "Everything done. It's all going in the place that goes in the place for each." Everything done, at last.

What a wonder it all is, that we appear and abide and fade away and no one knows what follows.

I WON'T FORGET YOU

INTRODUCTION

I won't forget you when you can't remember me.

I will remember everything.

I will remember for us both.

I will remember who you were.

I will remember who you have become and what that means for you.

I will somehow forgive what I said I never would.

I will remember to cry, deep and long and hard.

I will remember to open the door to your world.

I will remember to not ask "why" to just accept "why not?"

I will remember that I can be angry, not at you, but the disease.

I will remember to remember what you gave me, even if I can only see it now that you are "gone."

I will remember to let others help us. Help you. Help me.

I will remember to look for and find my own private joy.

I will remember that you have not forgotten the things that matter most.

I will remember that you have not, cannot, and never will leave me.

I will remember to see your face in mine.

I won't forget you when you can't remember me.

AUNT ADDIE
MALAIKA ADERO

Aunt Addie was already old when I was a young one, living in my grandparents' home. She was a member of the first generation of my family born free, in 1884. Her father migrated to their Knoxville home from middle Tennessee where he was enslaved, before he enlisted in the Union Army in his early twenties at the start of the Civil War.

Aunt Addie and her younger sister, Carrie, studied at Knoxville College, one of the many schools throughout the South founded at the end of Reconstruction for African Americans. Both girls were active in the African Methodist Episcopal Zion Church as missionaries. Carrie married a man who worked as a porter on the railroad, and Carrie, Addie, and Carrie's husband lived together and shared in the care of their father as he grew older. Addie was a businesswoman who worked from home as a seamstress. She was known not only for her fine custom work but for her own designs, particularly dresses with handkerchief tip hemlines. But when I was a child, the family said that Aunt Addie had "lost her mind." I know now that Aunt Addie suffered from a brain disease, and that disease was dementia.

She lived an independent life well into her middle age, but life took its toll on her health. So, she lived in the extended family household of her nephew and his wife, where she had a room of her own where she mostly kept to herself, speaking rarely. She kept her own counsel, read the Bible and tended to the Biblical objects in her tiny room: a bottle of Holy Water, an olive branch. These were souvenirs brought to her from the Holy Land, Israel.

I was the youngest—and arguably nosiest—member of the household, into everything and everybody but especially Aunt Addie. She was a great and compelling mystery to me. But she didn't talk much. She came out with us to have her breakfast, which always began with a tea cup of hot sugar water that she'd sip on for the longest time. She ate regularly but in small portions. And seldom said more than a complete sentence.

I watched her at the table, sipping sugar water. I watched how she ever so precisely folded laundry, smoothing the cloth with the flat of her hands, folding to 90-degree angles, flattening clothes and linens to stack neatly away until the cycle of use began again. Her skin hung from her bones like crushed velvet, wrung out while wet and left to dry without an iron. They said it was because she was once a stout woman who lost a lot of weight too fast. The irises of her eyes were ringed with a blue halo.

She spoke with her eyes and gestures. So, despite her strangeness, I was never afraid of her. I'd be shooed away by grownups, mostly to save her from the aggravation of my mischief. But, sometimes she did have what we called spells.

Aunt Addie would take off her clothes and replace them with strips of white cloth she collected. She'd tie them to her ankles and wrist. She'd come of out her room naked as the day she was born except for the white rags, and she'd run outside if not headed off at the door by my grandparents or some other adult. She didn't appear as old and frail as she usually looked when she pushed against them, trying to break free.

We didn't have neighbors in those days. So, there were no concerns about privacy. But we did have a lake out back that she might slip into. We lived on the lakeshore of property where my grandfather worked—Eastern State Mental Hospital. Our family had a long history with this hospital, which we called "the Asylum." My grandfather was a baker and butcher there, succeeding his father, who was a baker. My grandmother worked as a cook there as well, and later on with the patients. But Aunt Addie stayed home with us. Hospitals at the time did little to actually treat mental illness or diseases of the brain, and they were more like places to warehouse burdensome people. The science of the brain was still a young field.

When I got old enough to ask what made Aunt Addie "crazy," the answers did more to confuse me than to make the reasons clear. Grownups would mumble in response that she never married and how she was "too smart." Aunt Addie, they told me, was a college grad who was always bragged about for the good grades she made in school. She had a man in her life once, but I was told "something happened."

Knowing what we know now, I believe that Aunt Addie likely had dementia brought on by aging. Back then, we believed it was something that some people got, others didn't, and there was nothing to be done. My great-grandmother, Mama Allie, who also lived in this extended family household, worked puzzles, did needlework. She kept her mind and body as active as she could for as long as she could. I was her travelling partner on her many visits to family and friends in rural East Tennessee from the time I was a toddler until my early teens. She was my joy and I hers. But she developed dementia too. Her spells weren't like Aunt Addie's. But she did make a pile of clothes, including her daughter's good winter coat, and set it on fire in the backyard. And I did find her on the front porch crying, she said, because she thought I was pregnant.

Hearing this, I began to cry at the idea that she would even think that. I was an eleven-year-old virgin. I had not yet kissed a boy much less done the worst thing, in those days, that an unmarried girl could do: have a child. That shook me up as much as anything. When my grandmother realized what was going on, she offered words of reassurance to me and to her mama, Allie. A cycle of age-related dementia was beginning again.

By the mid-1960s, Aunt Addie's body weakened. She could no longer do anything for herself, so she was admitted to Eastern State. We had by then moved from the hospital grounds onto family land a short walk away. She was close, but so certainly away from us. My grandfather Lavon, her nephew, still worked there and could watch out for her on a daily basis. I was now a teenager, spending more time with my friends at school and home than with my elders. But I felt the growing distance between us all. And Aunt Addie was now like a phantom limb whose presence was felt even once she was gone.

MY MOTHER'S MIRROR
CATHY ALTER

I was prowling the aisles of my favorite consignment shop in Georgetown when the assistant manager, a friend, pulled me aside. Using the kind of voice reserved for men who pull open their coats to reveal a collection of stolen watches pinned to the lining, my friend said, "I have something to show you in the back."

She disappeared through a side door and returned with a small garment bag, which she unzipped slowly, like a burlesque dancer's slow reveal. "Tah-dah!" she said, as the garment bag fell to the ground.

To say it was a leather jacket would be an absurd understatement. What appeared on the hanger was more like a piece of high art, perfectly shrunken, seamed and shaped, with gunmetal rhinestones encrusted down the placket. All the Anna Wintours in the world could not have conceived of something this tough, this delicate, this perfect. Stepping closer, I noticed the label: Givenchy. As in Hubert de, the monsieur who put the H in haute couture.

"Is it a million dollars?" I asked, removing the jacket from its hanger and slipping it on. It certainly felt like a fortune, lined in silk and with sewing so fine it looked like China's "forbidden stitch."

"It fits!" cheered my friend, clapping her hands together.

"How much?" I asked, heading into the bathroom to look at myself in a mirror.

"For you," said my friend., "a hundred dollars."

A Givenchy for a Benjamin? I could definitely pull that off. I imagined all the places me and this jacket would go together, how transformed my life would be with this thing on my back, how velvet ropes would part, how photos would be taken, how autographs would be signed.

And then I saw how I looked in the mirror. With my son Leo at home napping and on my husband's watch, I had dashed off to the shop without showering or swapping my pull-on pajama bottoms for anything resembling real pants. My hair was a rat's nest, my face an oil slick. And even though I was wearing this amazing Technicolor dreamcoat, it was merely paper on an old fish.

I slunk out of the bathroom, bumping right into Alan, the store manager, who sized me up and down and delivered his verdict. "You need a better bra," he said coolly. "And for God's sake, put on some lipstick."

Handing the jacket back over to my friend, I didn't hear his biting commentary. Instead I heard my mother's, despite the fact that she hasn't spoken a clear sentence in years. Across the miles, from DC to a nursing home in Connecticut, she still holds up the most powerful mirror, whether I choose to look in it or not.

Although she is still alive, at seventy-two, she suffers from a progressive form of dementia that has robbed her of speech and, even more painful for me to witness, the ability to dress herself. For over forty years, as owner of our town's hippest fashion boutique, she told everyone within earshot how to dress, her daughter included. No longer in her trademark Love That Red nail polish and Armani black pantsuit, she sits locked in her head and strapped in a wheelchair, most days in sweatpants and with hair that's braided off to the side, which may be a convenience for her aides but surely is doing no favors for my mother. If she could return to her right frame of mind for even an instant, she would scream bloody murder. And then reach for her lipstick.

So how am I to keep up appearances? I am essentially without a mother and all the advice (solicited and un-) this title implies. For the past four years, I haven't had her to remind me to "floof" my hair (which, when I don't, makes me look like I have, her term, "cradle cap"). Nor is she available to tell me not to stoop ("you'll get a hunchback"), not to wear pale lipstick ("you'll look like a cadaver"), and not to wear boxy shoes ("you'll look like you have club feet").

And since Leo came into the picture, I am painfully aware that so many of us women who have kids later in life are motherless at such a significant time. It's a uniform I wear daily, even underneath the most beautiful leather jacket on earth (which incidentally, my mother would have berated me for leaving behind).

On days when I want to know about my own infancy, if I, like Leo, disliked green beans as a baby or how old I was when I stopped napping, I think: how can I do any of this without her? It's harder to imagine the bigger losses—the fact that she won't be at Leo's wedding, as my grandmother was at mine. Or that she won't be able to offer Leo a rare glimpse into his mother's past. She won't have the distinct pleasure of telling Leo stories about his mother when she was his age, the same kind of stories I had loved to hear about my own mother's precious girlhood.

Although I'm close to my father, I don't look to him for information. (The first and only time my father was left in charge, he attempted—and failed spectacularly—to teach my brother, who was two, how to change his own diaper.) He doesn't remember when I took my first step or spoke my first word. And when I asked him if he remembered how old my mother was when she went through menopause, the long hallway I'm about to walk, he looked like he was going to have a coronary.

Lately, I've been leaning on Joan, my mother's best friend, who reminds me so much of my mother with her candidness, her bawdy sense of humor, and her bootstrap sensibility. After receiving Alan's dry appraisal at the consignment shop, I emailed her and told her I was feeling a little sorry for myself.

"Pour yourself a drink, put on some lipstick, and pull yourself together," she wrote back, stealing a line from Elizabeth Taylor though she may have well been quoting my mother.

Still, I felt unable to obey their marching orders. For weeks I mooned about, agonizing over whether to buy the jacket yet not having the heart to march back to the shop—in my tired ol' pajama bottoms—and purchase it. I questioned whether I deserved something so chic when I had only the stroller brigade and early-bird diners at

Ruby Tuesday to impress. My glory days were behind me, and there were no guarantees of what lay ahead.

Then my birthday arrived, and my husband, the patient recipient of all that agony, presented me with a large box. I don't need to tell you what was inside, but I will tell you, when I saw it, I was stunned into action. An hour later, after fixing my hair and applying some red lipstick, I slipped on the Givenchy and insisted we hit the town. It's exactly what my mother would have done.

SISTER TRAVELERS

MIRIAM DeCosta-Willis

I knew something was wrong when I saw old newspapers stacked in front of her door, unopened presents piled under the dining room table, and the faucet running continuously in the flooded basement. Three months earlier, I had retired, intent upon writing books and hanging out with friends in Washington, where I had lived for a decade. I realized, however, that my mother needed help, so I decided to spend two or three days in Baltimore every week to take her to medical appointments, assist with her finances, and get the house in order.

I look back on that time, between the first signs of her health problem in late 1999 and her death in 2008, with mixed feelings: grief and guilt but also great joy and gratitude. I grieved for the mother— the funny, adventurous, courageous woman—whom I once described in an essay. But reading through my journals, I also remember the guilt that I felt for my impatience, bossiness, and failure to bring her to live with me. Instead, I rationalized that my lifestyle was too hectic for Mother in her declining years, because of my travel abroad and frequent trips to Memphis.

At times, I was exhausted by the caretaking: cooking, cleaning, doing laundry, paying bills, balancing checkbooks, handling unreported tax returns, and renovating the house. Mother once turned to me in anger and exclaimed, "You're killing me! Things are too rushed." Sometimes, I had to laugh at the two of us, who were so much alike—independent and stubborn women, determined to have our own way. For example, I threw out trash bags filled with old dishes and rundown shoes but, when I turned my back, Mother brought all her "precious stuff" back into the house. I outfoxed her, though, once I caught on to her game. I took those bags back to Washington and dumped them in the trash can there. Another time, a truck driver came, at my request, to take away old furniture from her damp, moldy basement. Mother didn't fuss at her caregiver (me!), but she yelled at the truck driver, "You're taking all my things! I'm going to call the police!"

The fall of 1999 was difficult for both of us, because it was a period of uncertainty and adjustment. Mother became increasingly forgetful and a bit "spaced out." She had little appetite, lost weight, and stayed in bed a lot—signs of depression. I suspected, too, that she was in the early stages of Alzheimer's, because she sometimes couldn't pronounce her words clearly and had a vacant look in her eyes. We were both familiar with the disease, because my stepfather had been diagnosed with AD, and Mother took care of him until she had to place him in a nursing home, where he died in 1998. In late September, my only sibling—and her favorite child—died suddenly in Albuquerque. Those two deaths, so close together, undoubtedly affected Mother's health. Meanwhile, I had five days to arrange my brother's cremation, write his obituary, and hold the memorial service, before leaving for Memphis, where my daughter was due to give birth. I was, thus, torn between caring for Mother in Baltimore and my family responsibilities in Memphis.

Eventually, I took Mother to a neurologist, who gave her an MRI, CAT scan, and psychological tests, which indicated that she did, indeed, have Alzheimer's disease. Later, I made an appointment with a medical social worker, because Mother refused to make long-term plans and I couldn't continue to commute between Washington, Baltimore, and Memphis. The social worker suggested that she move into a residence for seniors, but Mother replied, "I'm not going to be able to get myself together until February or March." She added that she was angry about my "interference" in her life, at which point I burst out crying and said, "Mother, I have to get you settled, so that I can get on with my eye surgery." Ironically, she became *my* caregiver when I had my first cornea transplant in January 2000. She was only in the early stage of Alzheimer's, so she was able to drive me to Johns Hopkins Hospital for the surgery and care for me at her home while I was recuperating.

When I was staying with her, Mother was more alert and animated, more compliant and appreciative of the attention. In one of her rare moments of reflection, she turned to me and said, "I hate to put you through all this." We spent evenings looking at family photos of Datie Mae and Uncle Boy, reading Daddy's love letters, and examining Grandpapa's property deeds. Those were moments of joy for both of us, because Mother told riveting stories about her family, as she recalled half-forgotten memories. She would begin, "Mama was a city girl from Atlanta, who thought Aunt Liza was a witch from Hancock County!" or she would ask, "Did I ever tell you about the letter Mama wrote to Spelman's president asking if they put saltpeter in the food?" We both laughed out loud, imagining Miss Florence Read's face when she opened the letter from my grandmother, Lillie Hubert. Mother's stories have influenced much of my research and writing, especially the book on my father, *Sojourn in Kaduna*. Growing up, I was a daddy's girl who declared, unabashedly: "I'm Papa's baby and Mama's maybe," but I became Mama's baby in the last decade of her life.

Over the next seven years, I moved Mother to senior residences in Baltimore, Silver Springs, and Washington, as she slowly declined, mentally and physically. She lost her vision, hid her Aricept pills, became more forgetful, and, eventually, was confined to a wheelchair. In her residences, we spent time together at musical concerts, chapel services, holiday suppers, visits with family, and parties with friends. She also enjoyed weekends at my Washington condo, Christmas trips to Memphis, and her ninetieth birthday party at the Radisson Hotel at Cross Keys. I learned to talk slower, listen more, stop rushing, follow her lead, and flow with her rhythm. For her part, she never, ever complained, even when we had to wait for hours at Dulles Airport because of ice in Memphis, spend the night in a motel, and get up at 4:00 a.m. to catch the next plane. Finally, I realized that we needed to be closer to family, so I moved back to Memphis in 2007, and placed her in a nursing home.

I wouldn't take anything for the experience of caring for Mother in her final years, because she, Beautine Hubert DeCosta-Lee—a social worker, college professor, and school administrator—taught me so much about love and life, aging with grace, and dying with dignity. Through moments of joy (sharing stories and laughing together) and moments of sorrow (her husband's illness and son's death), we became closer, sister travelers on life's journey. I have a memory of my mother to inspire and sustain me. Ironically, in the late 1990s, before we knew that she would soon be diagnosed with Alzheimer's disease, she testified before the Maryland State Legislature, as a member of the League of Women Voters, to request more funding for Alzheimer's research. In death, she passed the baton to me. So, in her memory, I joined the 2017 Memphis Walk to End Alzheimer's and raised money to help find a cure for that devastating disease. On that day, I walked in memory of Beautine Hubert DeCosta-Lee. And I walk every day in her memory because she was my mother, my sister, and my friend.

WALKING IN FAITH

An Excerpt from *On Pluto:*
Inside the Mind of Alzheimer's

COLLEEN (O'BRIEN) EVERETT

"Now faith is confidence in what we hope for
and assurance about what we do not see."
—Hebrews 11:1

Faith is a stretch at times. It is believing in something one cannot see, desperately reaching out at times into a void. Faith is the only thing stronger than fear.

My father has always been a man of faith. Some of my earliest memories of him are watching him kneel by his bedside with eyes closed, clutching a tattered Bible that was peppered with personal notes in his scratchy handwriting. A perfectly imperfect man, by his own admission, he would be so deep in thought and prayer that he would never even hear you enter the room. At the time, I was too young to understand the worries weighing on his heart, but I grew up learning that when life is difficult, or even when it is wonderful, or when one sins, as my father can with the best of them, one needs to close one's eyes and talk to God.

Everything was less scary to me as a kid, and eventually as an adult, because I saw the power of faith through my father's eyes: that no matter what life puts in front of you, God is already one step ahead of you. The Lord has a plan.

Well, I'm pissed off today about God's plan for my dad. Yet, I try in faith to listen.

Looking back, I don't ever remember my father yelling in torrents. He hardly ever lost his cool. When he coached my youth softball team, he would gently guide me to focus on fly balls instead of picking dandelions in centerfield with my childhood friend Liz Seymour. Or when our team cheered wildly after a member of the opposing team hit a home run—anathema to my sports-minded father—he would just smile. Or when as young kids, my brothers, Brendan, Conor, and I found ourselves on Saturday mornings playing hide and seek beyond stated boundaries by the printing press at the *Cape Codder* newspaper where Dad was editor and publisher, my father jokingly would get on the public-address system and loudly announce: "Brendan, Colleen, and Conor, to the principal's office! Brendan, Colleen, and Conor, to the principal's office!!"

Later, when I began dating, Dad welcomed boyfriends into the house with a hug instead of an intimidating glare. My older brother, Brendan, often had to take on the responsibility of scaring off rogue teen suitors. Dad rarely swore in front of us then, and treated everyone with respect; he saw the good in everyone—no matter their story, their look, or their past. Still does. He has always been one to reach out in gut instinct to help and mentor those in need, usually outside of the view of others.

Today is a different narrative in our journey with Alzheimer's. Now Dad has violent outbursts and eruptions of profanity. When he gets confused, which is often these days, he lashes out—usually at the people who love him the most. Outings with him can become uncomfortable, painful actually. At times, for example, I want to grab the waitress or cab driver, or whoever he's yelling at, and let them know it's not them, it's not him. It's Alzheimer's.

A few years ago, my father was invited to speak in San Francisco. The trip happened to coincide with my spring break as a teacher in Baltimore, so I agreed to go as his caretaker. He doesn't travel alone. I remember my mother asking if I was sure I could handle it. Living then several hundred miles away from the Cape, I didn't get to witness the full picture of my father. When he only saw me for a short period of time, he was able to use up all of his energy to be in the present with me. I didn't always see the darker side of the disease that my mother and brothers did. Until I spent a week as his caregiver, I had no idea how much of my father this disease has consumed.

Going through airport security without a second thought, I took my shoes off, put my bags on the conveyor, and walked through the AIT machine. I then heard someone spewing profanity behind me, and my stomach dropped. My father couldn't figure out how to take his belt off, and the TSA officer wouldn't let him through until he did. In that moment, nothing made sense to my father. He knew that he should be able to take his own belt off, yet couldn't. From thirty feet away, I had to watch the man who raised me to be a kind soul and taught me to field ground balls break down over his belt, as crowds of people stared in judgmental confusion over his confusion. In that moment, we switched roles. I became the parent. I closed my eyes, and asked the Lord for the strength to calm my dad. I made eye contact with him from the other side of the security screening, and coached him through the rest of the security line, like I would with one of my young students. I felt embarrassed and then immediately guilty for feeling that way. I knew that it was Alzheimer's, not my father. But that's the thing with Alzheimer's; it strips the person you love of all elements that make them who they are. There are many things that define my father—he is a devoted husband, a loyal friend, a loving father, an avid sports fan, and a stubborn Irishman. Alzheimer's does not define my father, but it does slowly strip away all of the things that do define him. All of the things that make him who he is.

My father today has become more childlike; the disease takes you there. And maybe that's a good thing toward the end of one's life. We all are so busy being adults that we forget the beauty and innocence of being a child, reinforced in me now as a young mother. Dad, in his disease, has found the balance sought in the Gospel of Matthew 18:2–4, "I tell you the truth. You must change and become like little children (in your hearts). . . . The greatest person in the Kingdom of Heaven is the person that makes himself humble as a child."

Dad is now a child in so many ways.

Each Father's Day, I can't help but wonder how many more I'm going to have left with my dad. And not just physically, but mentally—where my dad remembers me, and remembers my daughter, Adeline. It's a terrible thought, but one I can't seem to get off my mind. Watching him slip away has been one of the most painful things I've ever had to experience.

While I can't help these thoughts from flooding my mind, I also think of the wonderful memories that I do have: baseball games in the front yard; father/daughter trips to Fenway Park; ice cream at the Smuggler; and summer walks on the Brewster flats on the Cape. My father coached my little league softball team; as school committee chairman, gave the commencement speech at my high school graduation and handed me my diploma; surprised me with a yellow lab puppy for my sixteenth birthday; and walked me down the aisle on the most important day of my life. Alzheimer's may take a lot from my family, but it will never take those memories away from me.

It's really incredible to watch my father with my infant daughter. It's a moment I wasn't sure if I would ever get to have. I've read that children can reach those in the throes of Alzheimer's at a deep emotional level—a level that most adults can't. That's the grace of being a child, for Adeline and for my dad. I've seen it in the way that Adeline looks at my dad. She looks past his temper and his confusion, and only looks at him with adoration and love. When she smiles, she smiles with her whole face. She can't help but be all smiles when she's with my father.

She is in awe of him, as I am, too.

My father today has a short commute to work. The path from our home's back deck to his writing studio on the Outer Cape is lined with broken clam shells that mark the path like airport runway lights as he comes in for a safe landing. He can't get lost there.

Halfway up the narrow path, at the base of an old oak tree, is a yellow Tonka toy truck, weathered with age. Conor and I used to play with it. The wheels are now off; the plastic toy truck has been parked by the tree in solitude for close to twenty years. Dad put it there as a memory of our childhood, not far from what he calls "Christmas Tree Heaven," a patch of woodland on our property piled with the bones of family Christmas trees from all these years of our childhood. My father is a sap, excuse the pun.

The yellow truck, angels, and the color yellow are driving forces in his life; they give my father great comfort. It brings him back in faith to an innocent time, to childhood, and to his own young fatherhood. On his way to the office, he religiously touches the top of the toy truck and says a prayer, as if to reassure himself that he has a past. We often quietly witness the exchange from behind the sliding door of the family room.

In Baltimore, which I now call home, my husband, Matt, and I discovered a little more than a year ago that "we" were pregnant. I was carrying the baby; and Matt was carrying me. I had always wanted to be a mom; it's been something I've looked forward to my entire life. But as I sat on the floor with our new yellow baby lab, Crosby, awaiting the test results, a crushing feeling of anxiety swept over me: I was anxious about having to leave my six-year-old students a third of the way through the school year; I was anxious about being a good-enough mother; I was anxious about giving my students, my husband, my child, and our new puppy all of me. How does one even do that? I was far more fearful about passing the Alzheimer's gene on to our child. I was scared that if I had the gene, like my dad, I'd leave my baby too soon.

I woke up early one Saturday morning a few weeks later, then almost twelve weeks pregnant, and decided to go for a run—a route I've been running since we moved to our neighborhood in Baltimore.

There is a house on my route where three young kids live. They're always outside playing with chalk or games in the yard, and when I'm running by or walking Crosby, they love to say hi. When I ran by the house early that morning, no one was awake yet, but something caught my eye. By the big tree on the front lawn was a yellow Tonka truck—just like the one we grew up with. I stopped, held my hand over it, and felt a rush of calm. Faith told me everything was going to be right in God's plan.

This past Christmas Eve, I introduced my healthy baby girl, Adeline, to my father, a moment I never knew I would have. He held my angel tightly, and they danced slowly, grandfather and grand-daughter. All was good in that moment. While we do not know what the future holds for all of us, I've come to understand that we can have faith in God's plan. No matter what you choose to believe in, a personal choice for all, I've learned in this trial that one needs to have faith in something.

I have renewed faith today in angels, and in yellow Tonka trucks.

THE ECHO OF LOSS
CLEYVIS NATERA

"Spirits wandered. . . . They stayed with their descendants
to guide them through life, to comfort them, sometimes to
scare them into waking from their fog of unloving, unliving."
—Yaa Gyasi, *Homegoing*

When the picture frame fell and shattered, I knew my dead father
had come to pay me a visit. Pacing around my living room, I'd been
staring at my Fitbit as it counted my steps all wrong. One step lost for
every three it counted. When the picture frame arrived in my house
a week earlier, my cousin handed it to me with great ceremony and
said it was a gift for my fortieth birthday. I stared at my father, jaw
unhinged. I hadn't seen a photograph of him in two decades. I hadn't
seen him in the flesh in nearly three. I purposefully stuck the frame
on the highest shelf, finding the wood planks too small, I forced it in,
reassured by the snug fit. My littlest one, only three years old, liked to
climb, grab, throw. My bigger one, five years old, like to draw, paint,
then scrunch any kind of paper into a ball. But no way they'd get to
Papi that high up.

My older sister, Shany, was doing my daughter's hair. When the
picture frame fell off the shelf and the glass shattered, her hands hovered above those two gorgeous hair puffs.

"He's here," she said.

"I know."

She went back to the hair, avoiding my eyes. "For you or for me?"

"He's definitely here for me."

I picked up the broken frame, relieved the picture was unharmed. On the floor, pieces of glass, both small and large, waited for my attention. Each piece touched had my fingerprint, and the lines formed a map of sorts, I didn't know to where.

* * *

The first few months after we arrived in New York City, I thought constantly about Papi. He'd moved out of our house on Valentine's Day, a day before we left the Dominican Republic, and I had no idea where he lived. I wanted to imagine his life without us and couldn't. All four of us left at once: any, Shany, the oldest of us, was fourteen, Linda was twelve, was ten, and Evelyn, my little sister, was eight. The thought of our absence from his life was inconceivable. As though he must not truly exist, not without us. Much in the way our new life seemed surreal, leaving the heat of the tropics that February day to be greeted a few hours later by the frigid cold of Manhattan. Where had the heat gone? The anticipation of this new life had been a shadow cast over all the years since Mami left. Soon, she'd said year over year, we'd be with her. None of us realized it'd always meant without Papi.

In 1988, people like us made international calls by going to a calling center. Charged by the minute, the calls had to be brief. Weeks after we'd gotten settled with family, when we finally made our way in to call Papi, we found a space about the size of the average corner bodega. The line stretched out the door, half way down the block—people had come far to reach home. Up until then, everyone around us looked different but mostly the same, sounded different but spoke the same. Here we were, staring at people whose skin was shades lighter or darker, who looked past us as the cold made their hips dance from side to side, palms rubbed palms, sounds coming out of their mouths unintelligible. Even those who spoke Spanish were hard to understand; accents alien to us still belied the longing we ourselves felt. That day, awed, I thought about all the words that existed on the planet, how they could cleave: bringing people together or apart.

Mami was working her twenty-four-hour job as a home attendant in the Bronx. My aunt Miriam, a teenager at the time, had volunteered to take us, and as her eyes scanned the block, intent on finding her boyfriend, I realized everyone yearned.

Inside, each wall was lined with small, tempered-glass phone booths. We made our way to ours. On the way, the expressions of the people around varied. Concern, elation, sadness, even joy on the faces of those clutching phones. Regardless of squinting eyes or pressed lips, all the people I saw that day had one thing in common, bodies perched forward, listening intently when they stopped speaking, hands outstretched, touching glass.

That first time I spoke to Papi, I was too shy to say much of anything. We'd only been gone a few weeks. When I last held a phone in my hand, the situation had been reversed. Whenever Mami called us, no matter what we were doing, everything stopped. That last time, we'd run to the nearby neighbor's who'd summoned us to hear Mami's voice. That last time, it had been blindingly hot, a drought weeks in, the dirt ground split open like the cracked heel of a foot. That last time, he gently pushed my shoulder, urging me to speak to her, to tell her what I'd learned in school. Now it was his turn to be on the phone, oblivious to the distraction surrounding us, no one on this side gently pushing us to make conversation. Three of us squeezed into the booth that time.

The phone in my hand was heavy. It smelled like someone's dried spit. Struggling to say something, anything, I focused on the things I couldn't say.

The four of us had been separated. Evelyn and Lindo were down on 139th street with aunts who lived in adjacent apartments. Shany and I were living in our grandmother's apartment, sharing the top bunk in a room that housed three other people. Mami had decided we wouldn't go to school until September, even though we'd arrived in mid-February. Each gray day longer than the day before. We saw Mami maybe once a week, most weeks not at all. I'd been nagged by a terrible thought as we made our way to the call center:—we might have been better off if we never left.

My tongue was dormant. The hot, stinky phone pressed against my ear. Everyone stared. I'd been left to go last.

"What did it feel like when you first walked outside?" he said.

"The trees are naked," I blurted. "The branches look like my arms."

He laughed loudly, from the bottom of his belly.

"Now all I can imagine is a tree made up of arms," he said. "Your imagination . . . I will have nightmares tonight."

My shyness didn't last long. Within weeks, I learned to prepare. In the silence that followed one conversation, a quiet space that preceded the next, experiences took on a certain weight. Electrical currents that never left? = light, light. Drinking cold water with abandon? = mass measureless in volume. I once turned the faucet in the bathroom and watched it run. Time a tub filling with water. Until small waves lapped over the lip, trickled down the sides to claw feet, to floor. Not until that wetness slipped under the doorframe, traveled to the hallway, did someone think to check on me. Oh, the endlessness. Oh, the abundance! The pressure from the toilet water alone, when I pulled that lever, sounded like the cascading water of La Toma, the local river in our town. If you kept pulling at the lever of that toilet and held your face in close proximity to the bowl, it sprayed. You're so nasty, my aunt Miriam said when she caught my face so close to it. Those things though, they were not heavy enough to share. Back home, electrical outages were a constant. Cold water, a luxury. Water at all, a privilege.

One day, while on an errand with my other aunt, Suni, we heard a rumbling under our feet.

"Have you seen the train?" she said.

I shook my head "no."

She held my hand hard and pushed-pulled me down the stairs to the 145th Street train station. Back then, there was a 1 and a 9. The silver metal was moving too fast to register much more than the wind that swirled, the deafening noise a beat that repeated, relentless.

That feeling carried me for weeks, and I replayed my surprise at how huge the noise, how light ricocheted from the metal in motion, too many senses activated at once. I practiced talking to Papi, how I would describe it, anticipated what he would say.

When we next spoke, I said it reminded me of the ocean.

"Because of the noise?" he said.

"No," I said. "My heart felt so big."

On the other end, silence. I could sense his smile, his approval.

In those early months, it was his absence between the calls that made me pay attention. I saved each meaningful experience like a fragile thing inside a plantain tree leaf, the kind that grew in our backyard back in the place we used to call home; yes, leaves big enough to cover my small frame. Now I was the leaf. I kept the memories warm until I spoke them aloud.

Mami did it! She got an apartment in the Bronx and one of her sisters agreed to live with us, since she'd only be able to afford it as long as she kept working twenty-four hours a day, all seven days of the week. The toll on her was formidable. She seemed gone even when she was sitting right next to us, absent as she gently caressed our faces. The weight on her had already curved her neck down.

Months passed. By then, what felt like losing two parents was less jarring, not so dissonant. When we finally got to school, there was no bilingual classroom. We were assigned to a regular English-speaking class. Each night, I went to bed and prayed I would wake up able to speak English. Rays of sun found me kneeling on the bed, shouting garbled sounds I hoped were words, while in my heart knew they were not. Noche tras noche tras noche. Noches turned into weeks turned into months, and still words uttered into the illuminated dust particles of dawn were nonsense. Heartbroken, I didn't share that with Papi. Too heavy, I thought. Until one phone call I couldn't keep it in. I told him about my prayers and how despite the prayers each morning my tongue refused to speak English. I was learning nothing, no matter how hard I tried.

"You'll learn English," he said. "You're my most intelligent."

I snorted. It wasn't true. I certainly wasn't his smartest kid. But the way he said it, I could tell he believed I would. He lied to me so I would believe I could.

Silence created a space hollow enough to be filled with whatever I chose to put in it. I learned that words mattered, that preparing to tell a story was one way to keep him with me, and when I finally got to share it a piece of me got to stay with him. His responses were always a comfort. Around our town everyone called him Licenciado, Ingeniero, terms meant to show respect for an educated person though he'd never gone to school past 8th grade. He'd earned the title because he was a mechanic at an engineering plant specializing in heavy machinery. Papi was responsible for fixing the vehicles charged with charting new roads in San Cristobál, our town, and beyond it, vehicles that ensured the earth stayed in place with a coating of asphalt, or cement, or concrete.

* * *

Once, my little sister and I tried to count Papi's children with our fingers. My right hand counted the four of us, plus the first one born dead. I figured the dead counted, too. We kept each finger stretched stiff when they became people, and used the tip of our nose to count the others. Three quarters of the way we ran out of names to count but knew there were more children left. A hand's worth more? In New York City, he had a contingent of children who once tried to convince him to travel abroad. Papi had been clear in his disdain. He would never leave his land. The majority of his kids were in Santo Domingo, a twenty-minute drive from where we grew up. Close enough we could have had a relationship, but all the mothers refused.

Mami readily admits when she decided on him, a man twenty years her senior, it was first out of the necessity to leave Abuelita's house, last out of affection.

See, in true Dominican fashion, Papi had been a world-class womanizer. The thumb of my left hand was my half-sister J, who lived in our same town, who was only months older than Shany. Papi wasn't faithful, even to Mami (at least not at the start). It's possible Mami didn't get a life partner much different than the other mothers got. But we got a different father than the other children got. I know this for sure.

It was evident in how he cared for us, cooked for us, cleaned the house when the maid Mami hired to make up for her absence was off. It was evident when Papi took us to visit Condesa, his last common-law wife (the one right before Mami).

The house sat on a quiet, narrow street in Santo Domingo, painted the deep green of a royal palm tree. The front porch was lined with rocking chairs, and the four of us quickly took over the space. Within moments of arrival, we complained that we were hungry, thirsty, bored. One of my half-sisters, whose grown children were older than us, got fed up enough to scream at him that day. There must have been something in his attentiveness, traveling alone with four kids and no wife, probably requesting we be fed and be given water to pacify the whine. Maybe it was how he let us climb over his long body, sit on his lap, pull his thick, black hair. Most likely it was how happy he was with us, how happy we were with him. Whatever it was, her anger, resentment overlapped, and soon she couldn't contain it.

"One day," she told Papi, "when you're old and need your ass wiped, none of them will be here to do it. We're the ones who are going to have to do it."

I have no memory of his response. I was so taken by her anger, her bitterness.

I wish I'd turned my gaze to witness his thoughts, an accusation so fraught it must have drawn a reaction. Because by the time he turned into what she thought was the best version of a father, one she'd obviously never had, his offering was wasted on children destined to leave him. All while her hand remained outstretched for alms. Her words of course, were a kind of curse, a prophecy that came true.

* * *

I only saw Papi once between the time we left him and the time he died. Mami could hardly afford the trip when we found out he'd had a stroke. Un derrame cerebral, everyone said, a phrase that literally means cascade in the brain but sounded instead like a great surge, an awesome spill. We found him in a small house, thin and shrunken. The girl who was looking after him that day stood away from us, staring curiously at me from a door frame.

"You are sisters," Mami said.

I could tell. We had the same face. We looked like him.

I stole glances at her too. Obviously older than me but by how much? I was fourteen years old, she looked to be no older than fifteen, maybe sixteen. Exactly how long did it take Papi to change his ways? Did he ever?

Papi spoke slowly and was mostly out of it for the few days we were there. His thick head of hair was mostly white by then, as he was nearing seventy years old. His strong, lean body had become wiry, fragile. But his eyelashes curved thick and black, the bridge of his nose was as prominent as ever. By the last day, he could stand on his own, and as we walked away from the small house, he stood in the doorway, body slumped against it, watching us go. There was such sadness in his face I kept looking back to make sure it was true until I bumped into whoever was ahead of me. Now I realize he must have known. He must have known that was the last time he'd see us.

After that visit, the calls became less frequent on our end, and when we did call we were told he was sleeping or tired or unable to come to the phone. But I needed to hear Papi's voice. When I had had enough, I made Mami walk with me to the call center. I wanted answers. Her steps were tentative and so slow. I stopped in the middle of the street, in front of the fish place next to the call center.

"What's going on?" I said.

"He isn't well," Mami told me.

Of course, he wasn't well.

"Listen," she said. "His memory is almost gone."

In the call center, the phone booths had gotten much smaller than they'd been years before, when we first arrived. Or maybe I'd gotten bigger. Mami said a few words into the phone and then left it dangling, waiting for me. When I sat on the small ledge, the glass in front of me was smeared with fingerprints. Why didn't the people clean it after each use? On the other side, another booth stood empty, its glass just as dirty as this one.

Papi's voice was the same, a smile in it like usual. Relieved, I chatted on about school, about my upcoming sweet sixteen party. I'd suspected Mami was exaggerating all along.

After a few moments, he was quiet.

"Papi," I said. "Are you there?"

He cleared his throat.

"Who is this?" he asked.

I told him it was me, pronounced my name slowly. Your daughter.

"I don't have a daughter with that name," he said.

"Yes, you do," I said, so quietly.

"I don't."

He grew agitated.

"I don't."

On his side, someone took the phone, hung it up.

Desperate, I pressed my hand flat against the glass, saw it haloed by those other fingerprints. All of us, trying to push through glass, touch skin. All of us, so far.

Mami opened the door and took the phone away from me, hung it up. She wiped my face, and took me by the arm. Outside, the sun kept shining, and kids chased each other down the street.

The next morning, on a crowded 1 train downtown, I thought about how Papi would never get to ride in a train. He'd never get to feel winter, or see what trees without leaves looked like. Whatever he'd passed down to me—cells that traveled inside my body, from bone to vein to heart—were in the train, inside my body. Wasn't he in me at that moment? Wasn't he in the train? Between Papi and me, I found only silence. The hollowness now filled me up, and no matter how hard I tried, I didn't know how to fill it.

It wasn't hard to start talking to Papi in my mind. I'd had years of experience preparing, anticipating, guessing his responses (mostly right). The only difference was that now there was no comfort at the end. The only difference was that now I spoke to him mostly in English, and in my mind, he responded in a language he never spoke.

My vocabulary doubled because of language. Tripled, then quadrupled because of a newly acquired reading habit. His language receded until it was mostly gone. Phone calls became painful. Yet, within me his voice grew crisp, loud.

When I decided to go away to college, I struggled to convince Mami to let me go. In our Dominican culture, it was unheard of to allow an unmarried young woman go off on her own. Then, I remembered the strength of Papi's logic whenever he spoke to my mother, and in imagining how he would have convinced her to let me go, I mimed the words I was sure he would have used in my defense. If she wants a different life, she has to leave home, he would have told her. He would have reminded her. That's what I said, and it worked.

In college, there was a slight nudge that pushed me toward the boys who wouldn't try too hard to persuade to do what I wasn't ready to do, boys who wouldn't hurt.

When I got home for Christmas break, I slept for days on end, eating like I hadn't eaten in months, remembering a hunger I hadn't felt since childhood.

When Papi died, a couple of weeks later, I was the last one to find out. It'd been four years since we'd last seen him, but everyone was worried about how I would react. Everyone thought I'd be unable to deal. Maybe because I loved him most?

Knowing he no longer occupied space in the real world was a stunning blow. There are no words to explain how the absence thickened, how this loss pressed on my chest, fractured bone, punctured lungs. Within days of his passing, when we realized there was no way to afford getting on a plane, there would be no goodbye, I noticed how from time to time the air around me took on a slightly different density, as it does when another reaches over to give a hug, thin air easier to breathe. I was being watched over. Nearly twenty thousand miles divided us, him now under dirt, yet I became certain Papi was with me, just as he'd been all along.

What method do the dead have to talk to us but through our

bodies? Since my father died, that hollowness turned into a dull ache in my bones. This ache is the silence between conversations, and I've learned to listen for what the silence holds. It is the force that binds us, that needs no tongue. But when I'm too stubborn to listen, picture frames fall.

Once, while wrapped up in a passionate affair, I dreamed we waited for my father so this lover could meet him. In this dream, we both knew he was dead, so it was especially important they were going to meet. My boyfriend made a flimsy excuse and left the meeting place. I'd been left with the uneasy feeling Papi was already there, looking at us from afar. In the morning, unsure what to make of it, I shared the dream with him. Sounds like a warning, he said. Things fell apart quickly after that. Whose shady intentions can stand up against that kind of protection?

I only visited Papi's gravesite once. The trip back home was the first thing I saved for after graduating college. Only three out of the four of us got to make it, since Evelyn had a small baby and was unable to travel. We were only a few feet away from his grave when Shany fell heavily over it. The raised tomb was a rectangle made of concrete, crowded on both sides by other people's dead. Shany's sobs shook her shoulders. I'd never known one set of eyes were capable of that many tears. Lindo, who'd been back in the Dominican Republic a few years by then, followed closely behind. He cried without restraint, without shame, whatever machismo he'd held onto forgotten. Eyes dry, I shifted from foot to foot. You're cold, Lindo said when we walked away. I nodded. The moment mired by reality. How could my father fit in such a small rectangle? What had they done so his body stayed bound, didn't break through the concrete? How could a giant be made to fit in a place meant for a human? That day, Lindo and Shany went to his grave to say a long overdue goodbye. But I wasn't there for that. As we walked away, I didn't once look back. Body lighter, my limbs lengthened; skin thicker, my bones hardened. Bienvenido Natera—my body is his final resting place.

UNFORGETTABLE

An Excerpt from *On Pluto:*
Inside the Mind of Alzheimer's

BRENDAN MCGEORGE O'BRIEN

Memory is a powerful thing. I think of it as a time capsule, protecting life's most unforgettable moments. It reminds me why I find comfort in hearing my dad's voice and joy in seeing his face. My memories of him paint a picture of the man who has been my lifelong hero, my mentor, and my best friend.

That's why Alzheimer's is terrifying; it leaves a menacing wake in its path. As my father's memory erodes, so too will his perception of who I am, who he is, and of every moment we've spent together.

It's a disease that has no compassion for what I hold closest to my heart, the memories I've shared with my dad. That's why the word *unforgettable* has new meaning for me these days.

Growing up as a salty local on Outer Cape Cod, it's a birthright to have a deep respect and appreciation for its natural beauty. The Cape has always been a special place to my dad, so of course, it became a special place to me. He never missed an opportunity to profess his love of its surroundings, and as a firstborn son, I was his sidekick in exploring its splendor.

One thing I'll never forget was watching the miles of magnificent coastal dune erode into the Atlantic Ocean. It felt like our home was slowly washing into the sea, one winter storm after another. I think that's why my dad cherished the Cape so much; he knew it wouldn't be there forever.

Years later, I learned that the sand washed out from those dunes would traverse miles down the beach, often forming into the perfect sandbars that I coveted as a young surfer. Dad's wisdom still rings true: "It takes time, but nature always finds a way to fight back," he'd say.

Almost 25,000 years ago, Lower Mill Pond in Brewster was just a lifeless crater discarded from the Laurentide Ice Sheet. The pond, long-sufferingly, had spent millennia transforming itself into a brilliant habitat, one of Cape Cod's historic kettle ponds. In childhood, it was a sanctuary to me, another place where my dad taught me of nature's unrelenting force and to marvel at its creation. We were fascinated by the herring that thrashed upstream in March to spawn, the spring leaves that grew back from a dark winter, and the pond that would thaw just in time for us to grab a canoe and explore. Nature's timing is perfectly flawless.

A couple decades later, I found myself sitting at the edge of that same pond. Skirting the tip of a large granite boulder, a remnant of the ice sheet, I sat quietly next to my father blankly staring into the distance. The crowds were gone, the air was light, and winter was just a few storms away. Just like the old days, but watching the autumn leaves drift in the wind and the flocks of osprey fly south, it felt different this time. A haunting silence loomed between us, our emotions bottled, ready to let fly. My dad had Alzheimer's and there was nothing left to say.

Earlier that day, I had signed his power of attorney documents, now becoming the guardian. Our sinking reality snapped into focus; it was finally time to let go.

Tears began streaming down my father's face, "I'm so fucking scared, Brendan," he mustered, "I don't know what's happening to me!"

Seeing him cry for the first time has burned itself into my memory. I remember wanting to tell him that it would be okay. But I couldn't. I knew it wouldn't be okay. So we buried our heads into each other's arms and sobbed, letting our fears of the unknown cascade into the pond. It was one of those unforgettable moments, and we shared it together.

We're often told the torment of Alzheimer's doesn't start in a nursing home—far from it. It's a journey that takes decades, starting long before your bags are packed. There is no map, no trail, no True North, just a destination that no one wants to reach.

In hindsight, our family had blissfully ignored the blatant warning signs. My dad's once "artistic quirkiness" and consummate presence was slowly transforming into an introverted, disconnected personality. He had always been the catalyst of a party, the kind of person everyone wanted to be around. But now he seemed alone, misunderstood. Life was a lot easier when we thought that was just part of getting older.

What we were never told was that a tsunami was heading our way and all we had was an umbrella. We found our shelter through empathy, doing our best to understand. My dad compared it to a surfer paddling out in the middle of a nor'easter—frantically using every ounce of energy to get beyond the sand bar, duck diving beneath a giant crashing wave milliseconds before it could wash you back to shore. But the second you come up for air, there's another one right behind it, pounding the sea in front of you. It's a draining battle where nobody wins. But the harder you paddle, the longer you'll last. I've learned that much from my dad.

The hardest part for me is that the story of our lives together, as a father and son, is slowly drifting away, one unforgettable moment at a time. From his first grandchild to the ones he'll never know, our first trip to Fenway Park, driving me to North Carolina for college, it all washes away. The memories erode. We start it all over again. Eventually, there is no such thing as *unforgettable*.

But if nature can find a way to heal, I think we can, too. Our journey with Alzheimer's has been filled with challenge, but it has also been filled with opportunity—opportunity to share our story, to strengthen our relationships, and to cherish the time we have left.

The war against Alzheimer's is one we can all wage together, but the only way to win is to talk about it, take it public and bring it out of closet. With more than 50 million afflicted across the world, we have power in numbers. Nothing will be done until local, state, and federal governments hear from the masses. So it's up to us. We'll never fully understand the disease until we collectively listen to the stories of those affected, the frontline. It's the truth, in our vulnerability, that will create real progress.

Mom, Dad, I'll always be right there with you guys, fighting dementia with all I have. Everything you've taught me will live far beyond our years, and I wouldn't trade that for anything in the world. Our love is what's truly unforgettable, wherever we may be.

BRINGING JOHN BACK HOME
DANIEL C. POTTS, MD, FAAN

"We want to stay with John. We are committed to him, and to preserving his story."

He wandered in reluctantly. A sky-blue windbreaker was the first we were to see of him and would be the last. (God must have used the same paint for his eyes.)

The steel-built Vietnam veteran stiffly entered the first art therapy session and sat with crossed arms and pursed lips at table's end. Two female student partners timidly took their places beside him and began the humbling and uncomfortable task of learning how to communicate with someone whose verbal skills were being lost to dementia. John had severe expressive aphasia, the loss of expressive language, though he retained most receptive abilities. Thus, he could understand what was being said, but had great difficulty expressing thoughts and feelings through words. His aphasia accompanied three other characteristic features of Alzheimer's disease: amnesia (memory loss), apraxia (inability to perform familiar tasks), and agnosia (inability to process sensory input).

"This may be challenging," I whispered to one of the students, out of earshot and eyesight of John. I wanted to encourage them, and to let them know I would be nearby to help.

As the art therapist explained the directive for the first session, it became apparent that John was not going to be making any art. At least, not the art that was called for in the directive. He spent most of the session coaxing his student partners to draw and cut shapes to place on a white paper background. Almost no words were understandable, but occasionally one could make out, "I need to do what I want to do," or "it has to come from in here," putting his hand over his heart.

A neurologist and the instructor for the course, I sat in the background observing, thinking how much John reminded me of my father; I wanted to go near and encourage him. To tell him I was proud of him (just for showing up for life) like Dad always had told me. I thought perhaps, at some level, he needed to know.

Dad's favorite color was blue. Sky blue. Like his own eyes. And John's.

My father, Lester, became a watercolor artist in the throes of Alzheimer's disease, having never painted prior to the diagnosis. Witnessing the expression of Dad's personhood through art completely changed my medical practice, as I grew in empathy, understanding, and hope to share with others on a similar journey.

After Dad's death, my family and I created a foundation, Cognitive Dynamics, with a mission to improve quality of life for persons living with dementia and their care partners through the expressive arts and storytelling. Our primary initiative was inspired by Dad's story and art: *Bringing Art to Life* pairs students with persons living with dementia. Each semester, students from diverse backgrounds develop friendships with their dementia partners, creating art together under the guidance of an art therapist, learning the life stories and character traits of their partners, and honoring them by creating leather-bound legacy books filled with art, letters from loved ones, important life events, and writings from the students. The program builds empathy in the students, lessening the stigma attached to dementia and aging, and promotes self-growth. It validates persons with dementia in their current state and gives respite to care partners.

Observing the development of these intergenerational relationships over the years has been one of the highlights of my career. Each semester has its relational gems. But none has affected me more profoundly then that of John and his two student partners.

John was a tough nut to crack, his hard shell impervious to most who tried to engage him. But I held out for that almost miraculous transformation I'd seen happen many times before, when the relational phenomenon finally unfolded through a space cleared by mindful listening, compassion, intention, and presence.

Sure enough, John started warming to his new friends. His body language became more open, and he began participating more actively in the art projects. In one very tender exchange after several weeks of art therapy, John reached over and touched the hand of one of his student partners, telling her she had done a good job with her art. Later that day as they escorted John out of the art therapy session, he told his student partners that they were "good people."

The breakthrough came the day musicians visited an art therapy session, playing and singing familiar songs for the students and their partners. By the end of the session, John was dancing with anyone nearby. He even came up and placed his arm around me, harmonizing with me on "Amazing Grace." This was a moment of deep connection which I feel at some level will never be forgotten. We witnessed John's spirit breaking through the shackles of dementia that day, singing and dancing its way into all our hearts. His students were profoundly moved by what happened in that room.

That was the last time we saw his blue windbreaker, blue eyes, blue soul. Two days later, John wandered away from home in the middle of the night. His body was found six weeks afterward in a ravine not far away.

When it became apparent John likely would not return to our program, I met with his students to give them options about how to finish the semester. Either they could stay with John, completing his life legacy book with information they already had garnered and impressions they had developed, or we could choose another partner for them with which to work over the remaining weeks. Without hesitation, both said they wanted to stay with John, to honor his personhood by creating the best legacy book possible for his family, and simply to express the gratitude they felt for the experience of working with him.

For the remainder of the semester, John's students centered themselves completely on the person they had come to know, interacting together within this personhood during each ninety-minute art therapy session. They reminisced while discussing John's unique character traits, and the impact he had made on them in a few short weeks. It was as if John, in all the deep blue of his selfhood, had sashayed right back into the room.

In one way, the finding of John's remains brought some closure for the students, as I am sure it did for his loved ones. But all of us must deal with the longing to sing and dance with him again, to build upon the relationships that had developed, to hear his wise, yet jumbled words, to wade into the blue pools of his eyes. Such a longing wells up alongside the pain of Alzheimer's, in our pain about the cruelty of this disease.

Alzheimer's is a thief; only death, itself, is its equal. But even Alzheimer's can't steal the essence of personhood or the beauty of relationships. Those live on through the power of love. In some essential sense, personhood is relational, and dependent upon those loving interactions that touch the core of who we are. And they develop in the broad and level space of presence: the ground turned holy by the vulnerability and authenticity of persons who choose to enter the reality of another without trying to control it, and without losing the integrity of their own personhood. That's what John's students did, and I am so proud of them.

I believe personhood is eternally remembered in the mind of God. We can be of the same mind.

Bringing Art to Life completes each semester with a celebratory dinner in which the students stand up and say what the experience has meant to them, honoring and validating their partners living with dementia. Though not physically present at this event, John was very much with us through the reverence and gratitude expressed as the students shared his story, and the transformation it had wrought in their lives.

In the end, they brought the wanderer back home through a friendship that reached far deeper than fractured phrases and fading memories, stretching clear across the divide of generations and disabilities, to a place where we all are one. I wonder if they know they brought themselves back home, as well?

There was another presence in the room at the celebration that night. If I am the only one who felt it, that makes it no less real. And Dad's eyes were beaming as big and blue as those of his new friend, John.

EIGHTY-THREE YEARS OF IMMORTALITY
Nihal Satyadev

It was not often that the corridors of a state-run hospital in Hyderabad, India, became crowded because of a singular patient, but this case was peculiar. Nurses and paramedical staff flocked beside the young patient who was writhing in pain, in an attempt to offer solutions. They were all left stumped. A young man, who had spent time in some marshlands near his village, was driven nearly a hundred miles to the city and brought to this hospital. A leech had lodged itself in his left nostril and was gorging at will. There was great concern of the leech inching toward the brain and potentially causing lasting damage. As the assigned doctors were discussing various options, Dr. Siromani Ananthula was passing by and inquired about the commotion. It took her only a few minutes to devise and implement a solution. Moments later, she was next to the patient with a candle in one hand and a bowl of water in the other. Strategically placing the two items above and below the nose respectively, she lured the leech toward the water and easily extracted it with forceps. Ultimately, this case would prove to be by no means her most difficult but rather one of the several instances over the course of her medical career where she was able to showcase her breadth of knowledge and ability to think quickly in volatile situations.

Siromani Dharmavaram (she would later change her name after marriage) is my grandmother and today, at the age of eighty-three, she has Alzheimer's disease. She was born in 1935, twelve years before

India gained its independence, in the town of Gooty in the Kurnool District of Andhra Pradesh. Her father was not only a respected senior official in the state education department but also earned the nickname "Panther Naidu" for his reputation of protecting nearby villages from big game—tigers and panthers that would often pick off small farm animals. It was later discovered his kill count well exceeded one hundred fifty. Her mother, as was common back then, bore the responsibility of raising the children. Her dedication to this effort would eventually manifest an inexplicable bond between her and her oldest daughter, Siromani.

As soon as Dr. Dharmavaram finished her medical education, she moved back home to Kurnool. For six months, she worked eighteen-hour days as a house surgeon. Immediately after, she was able to start her own general medicine private practice, having gained the trust of her community through her exceptional bedside manner and medical skills. Within a year after that, she was appointed as the medical officer of the Kurnool District and then to the state medical service. Even today, nearly fifty years later, the people of Kurnool still remember her services to their family members.

Soon after, with the blessings of her parents, she married a young police officer, Venkat Rao Ananthula, a rising star in the police force. Like Siromani, Mr. Ananthula also came from a lower-middle class family. He, too, developed an impeccable work ethic during his youth, maintaining a job as a railway clerk during the day while putting himself through college during the night. It was amid his first year of college that he took and passed the Andhra Pradesh State Civil Service Exam and was selected among thousands for one of three openings as the deputy superintendent of police.

During the early years of marriage, Dr. Ananthula would move often as her husband's postings ranged from fighting Chinese forces in the northernmost parts of the country to protecting one of the most sacred temples in Southern India. It was only a few years later that they were able to settle in the city of Hyderabad.

In June of 1969, Hyderabad was rocked with violent riots. Hundreds of thousands of people took to the streets and several police officers wound up in the emergency rooms of various hospitals. As one doctor was about to treat one of these trauma-stricken young officers with a dose of penicillin, Dr. Ananthula rushed in to stop the doctor, ordering him to first administer a test dose to rule out allergic reaction. Through this swift action, she saved the life of the hyperallergic young officer, who happened to be none other than her husband.

Mr. Venkat Rao would spend the next decades rising to the highest ranks of the state's police force, and Dr. Ananthula, too, would go on to blossom in her career. She studied and acquired further degrees that allowed her to specialize in Ophthalmology and quickly rose to the Head of Ophthalmic Surgery at one of the largest hospitals in one of the biggest cities in the country.

While my grandmother, or Ammamma *(umm-umm-ah)* as I call her, had an illustrious career, her true character was reflected in the role she played within the family. At a young age, she realized the difficulties her mom was enduring to raise her and her five siblings. Ammamma was committed to doing everything possible to help her mother. Over her first fifteen years as a medical professional, a majority of her earnings would go towards funding her siblings' education and marriages. She, personally, found more satisfaction in seeing the family succeed than in her own success. At the time, during her early career, this was by no means a small economic sacrifice. Dr. Ananthula neither allowed herself to get her own vehicle nor ever spent money on developing any hobbies. Raising her siblings as a second mother, she would ensure that they all became either doctors, dentists, or teachers. It was only because of her tremendous efforts that her siblings all went on to be financially stable. For nearly two decades, Dr. Ananthula would balance being a full-time doctor, a mentor and provider for her siblings, and a mother to my own mom and her younger brother—three roles that required massive investments of time and love.

Ammamma played a big role in my upbringing as I would often spend summers with her during my earliest years of formative development. Growing up, I neither knew the stature Ammamma had in the community nor the depth of knowledge she possessed in the medical field. All I was acquainted with was the unending efforts she took to ensure I was well cared for. She would read to me every night, implement master strategies to feed the picky eater I was, and share her love for classical music through impromptu karaoke nights— anyone who can bear my screeches and convince me they are song is already a hero.

Many in my family considered her to be a wonder woman, but Father Time would ultimately prove them wrong. In 2011, after already having had a few years of cognitive decline, my grandmother was officially diagnosed with Alzheimer's, and her role at this point in the family began to change rapidly and precipitously. However, her lifelong compassion to her family and her community is not one that is forgotten. This love continues to live on through my grandfather, who tirelessly provides her with comfort and care through the progression of the disease, and by the inspiration she has been for me to live out her example through my own life. When I visit my family in India, I see a woman who is a beacon of integrity and compassion.

A few years ago, I began volunteering with the Alzheimer's Association to advance policy efforts and lobby members of Congress. My role required that I analyze census data to create demographic fact sheets for each congressional district in Southern California. As I scrutinized the projections, I recognized that the cost of care for those with Alzheimer's was on a trajectory to bankrupt the US healthcare system within a couple decades. This was clearly a concern for my generation. As an undergraduate, I was shocked to learn that there was no national organization working to inspire students in fighting for this cause.

This was the impetus to found my nonprofit, The Youth Movement Against Alzheimer's. My mission was to rally students to source solutions by addressing this as the public health crisis of our generation—to create and grow a nonprofit that I feel reflects the creativity and compassion of my grandma. In a few years, we grew to actively engaging over five hundred students, each with their own connection to the disease. We support caregivers like Hannah, a high school senior in Alabama who cares for her single mom who has early-onset Alzheimer's. For young people like Hannah with no other access to community support, the Youth Movement Against Alzheimer's serves as an extended family.

One of the nonprofit's most critical successes was the creation of a low-cost respite care model. With 40 percent of family caregivers for persons with dementia suffering from depression, a breakthrough respite care is among the most needed support for family caregivers. The pairing of trained student volunteers and persons with dementia for just six hours a week yielded significant reductions in self-reported stress for family caregivers. As the program scales to other campuses, we have the opportunity to inspire more students to enter the fields of aging and save the healthcare system billions by delaying entry into assisted living facilities and nursing homes. By serving as one of the volunteers myself, I was able to get a deeper appreciation for the elderly. I was paired with seventy-four-year-old Richard, and we would find ourselves lost in conversation as he regaled with tales of his career in academia. Weeks later, his wife told me, "Nihal, you are the reason Richard has a purpose again—he's happy." Ammamma would be proud.

As our nonprofit continues to reach more students and shape policy efforts to address the growing national and international aging and care crisis, I remind myself of the life my grandmother has lived thus far. Ultimately, it is her values of compassion to family and community that we need to foster as a country in order to solve some of our most difficult healthcare challenges. *Ammamma,* you are evergreen in our memories. Your legacy will continue to live on through me and the millions we hope to inspire.

TYING ALAN'S SHOES
WREN WRIGHT

I'm waiting for Alan to get dressed. It's the first day of autumn, and we're taking a day trip to the mountains. He finally appears, calmly proclaims he can't tie his shoes, would I do it for him? He's had difficulty dressing himself. This morning he was able to pull on his socks and pants, button his shirt, and pull a sweater vest over his head.

Alan and I have been married for three years. I'm fifty-seven, he's sixty-five. He was diagnosed with dementia nine months after we recited our wedding vows. It's the second marriage for both of us, but the bond between us is fierce. With wet eyes, envious friends have told us this kind of love is rare, that we live in a dreamy fairy tale. We think it's enchanting and perfect.

This dementia, the thief, takes its time fracturing our union. No one and nothing but this wretched disorder pulls us asunder.

Today we'll drive to our favorite mountain town, and we'll promenade along the Riverwalk, for this is the extent of Alan's dwindling capabilities. No more off-trail or dirt path hiking. We stick to boardwalks and paved pedestrian routes. We'll walk upriver holding hands the entire time, like always, staggering toward the future. We'll take in the crisp, dry air and watch the wind rustle through the pine and aspen trees.

We'll visit the stationery store where we'll buy journals that have fancy leather covers and pages edged in gilt. We'll carry them close to our hearts while we amble downriver to our favorite coffee shop. Then we'll sit at a black wrought iron bistro table on the outdoor patio, listen to the moving water, watch passersby as we sip chai and munch hazelnut biscotti. We'll transfer the pain of losing each other onto the lined acid-free pages of our new books, trusting the journals and the rushing river to assimilate our words and emotions into our souls, somehow making sense of it.

At dinnertime, we'll saunter upriver to our favorite Italian restaurant where we'll have a glass of Chianti and a bowl of bow-tie pasta with pesto sauce. Then at dusk, we'll follow the river to a wooden bench under a stand of aspen trees, the perfect vantage point to watch the deer coming down from the forested hills for an evening snack, unfazed by our presence on the other side of the water.

Then finally we'll drive home, snaking down the mountains and foothills, on the lookout for feeding elk and perhaps a herd of mountain goats. We'll smell the heady wood smoke rising from nearby chimneys and hold hands that much tighter, present in each other.

At home, we'll speak softly of how lucky we are to have found each other. Then we'll fall asleep in each other's arms, dreaming the same dream of floating downriver, wishing it could always be this sweet for us, wishing the thief had knocked on someone else's door.

Alan wakes me from my thoughts, plants a warm kiss on my cheek, adding a dash of playfulness he sometimes mixes into our private moments. He plunks himself down on a dining room chair, his arms resting on its arms. He points to his unlaced, polished brown Rockports, bringing me back into the present.

I descend to the floor, touch his leg to steady myself, bend over his feet, lift the ends of the laces on his left shoe and cross them to begin the tie. It's an ordinary, simple action.

Or so I think.

I become dizzy and nearly lose consciousness as I slip into a different knowing. In an instant, a brilliant flash of white light penetrates my skin and slides into every cell of my body. It takes over subtly, moving my hands and fingers. *It's not me tying my sweetheart's shoelaces—it's this mysterious force, full of light, love, generosity. I'm merely its catalyst. I imagine I'll swell to accommodate it, but I don't. Rather, it seeks release through my actions.*

What an honor to tie Alan's shoes!

As I form each bow and finish each tie, I sense the absolute *purity* in this ordinary act. *Alan's shoelaces are the medium and I am the conductor.*

This force, which I can describe only as love and its infinite nature, streams through me again and again, and I am in bliss. *This is where the sacred resides—in performing an unpretentious task mindfully. And again a wave of reverence passes. A privilege to tie Alan's shoes!*

I move to his right foot, the love within me expanding. *This is the love that moves the universe. It's the love at the heart of our being, and that love is simply all there is. When our fears and worries and emotions are stripped away, it's love and only love that remains.* When Alan cannot tie his shoes, it's love that asks me to do it for him, and it's love that complies.

Although my revelation began meekly with an uninspiring task, *this love is the force that encourages us to live fully in the mundane.* It's the force that loves and animates Alan and me and each one of us. It's the force that loves shoelaces and the rhythm that marks our days.

I finish tying my husband's shoes, rise from my place at his feet, and suddenly I understand that the day I will not tie Alan's shoes is the day he will not need them. It's the day he'll leave his shoes behind, the day he'll leave this world. I wipe a tear from my eye, grateful that I am the one to tie Alan's shoes.

I rise from the floor. We gather our things and load into the car, back out of the garage, and drive toward the mountains. Today we have a river to cross.

SEALED AND DELIVERED
Wren Wright

It's midafternoon and the soft, full northern sunlight creeps into my husband's hospice room. He lies motionless in what's been his bed the past fourteen months. His hands are folded across his chest, the way he often slept the entire time we were together. I always wished he wouldn't sleep in that position. I couldn't bear what it foreshadowed.

He breathes in short, quick bursts, like a majestic being giving birth to the universe, powerful and joyful in its progress and pain. Alan has not been responsive for nearly twenty-four hours now. Dementia has finally won. His nurse says he's in the active dying process, that the end will arrive long before the morning comes.

I sit with him for the last time. I hug him and speak softly to him, although I don't know where I find my voice, and I don't know if he knows I'm here. Surely, he must. I kiss his hand, his cheek, his mouth, and whisper my love to him, offering it as a guide, a line I hope he'll carry into the next world.

I dab water into his mouth like the hospice nurse showed me. I read to him. When I lose my voice and run out of words, I silently ask for guidance and am moved to be still, to be quiet, to maintain a calm presence. I hold his hand and remember our life together. I run my hand up his arm and feel the electricity between us—the energy that's always been there, the essence of us as one being. I'm empty, my mind uninhabited.

Rebecca, the hospice chaplain, floats into the room carrying the spirits of all who have walked this path before. She embraces me, passing along their understanding and strength. Rebecca is no ordinary chaplain. She's an ordained minister who also does spiritual. Alan and I claim holds on no religion, but we do spiritual.

I sit on my husband's right side, Rebecca slips in on the left. She opens a vial of oil. Anointing rose oil, she tells me. She takes Alan's pale left hand in hers, pats it softly. She dips her index finger into the oil and gently traces on his palm, dabbing first in the center of it, then spreading the oil in a circular motion, slowly spiraling to the exterior of his upturned hand. When she's done, she reaches out for mine. I offer my left, and again she dips her finger into the oil. She traces the same spiral on my palm. I'm nearly breathless but present and open to what's about to happen in this impromptu ceremony.

"The spiral," Rebecca begins, "is an ancient symbol found in almost all cultures throughout the world. The spiral is visible throughout nature. We live in a spiral galaxy. Behold the helix shape of our DNA spirals, the spiral shape of the hurricane, the tornado, the nautilus shell.

"Our lives mirror the form of a spiral. Life is a cycle of birth, growth, death, rebirth. However, we don't experience life as a circle, we experience it as a spiral. We learn, grow, evolve, always returning to the same place, but with more experience and knowledge than before. This spiral journey makes our world larger. Our perception has changed and we can face the same sort of situations we did before, this time with a fresh perspective. This opens new pathways, new ways of seeing and being. The entire process is thus put into motion again and again, life spiraling perpetually from inward to outward."

My soul knows this, even if I don't, and I want to hear more. I long for tales of the spiritual journey and how my sweet husband and I will live on together, forever.

Rebecca puts my left hand in Alan's left hand. She holds them together, pressing our spiraled palms each into the other, mingling the anointing oil, melding the essence of the rose oil from his hand into mine, from mine into his. He's still unconscious and unresponsive but alive and aware, I'm convinced, at a level just out of reach yet present enough.

"As the spiral symbolizes both cosmic and earthly forces, so the spirals I've drawn on your palms represent your lives together on the spiritual plane as well as here on the physical. Know that both of you, Alan and Wren, are bonded together throughout time, just as strongly as you are attached here on Earth. Nothing and no one can separate you. This cosmic connection between the two of you is invisible, yet its strength is more powerful than any earthly betrothal. Its underlying strength is love, and love is indestructible. Love is the foundation of all things and is the only thing."

I'm fully present, hanging on every word Rebecca speaks. Alan's hand and mine are still joined together, and I can't tell whose hand is whose. His breathing pauses as a regal smile overtakes him.

From deep within me yet right in front of me, I hear Rebecca. "Alan and Wren, the universe recognizes you to be husband and wife for all eternity, never beginning and never ending, together forever."

I gasp and let out a muffled cry at what's taken me these last minutes to realize. This ceremony on Alan's deathbed, more precious now than our wedding ceremony, unites us for all time, through the ages, not just on earth.

I'm in a sort of trance, hearing only a whirring sound in my head, watching my husband, seeing only him. I don't notice when Rebecca slips out of the room. I sit awhile, holding Alan's hand, pressing our spiraled palms together, wanting to hold him forever, to walk with him side by side, to fly away with him.

Outside it's grown darker, quieter, calmer. I'm still at Alan's side when the sun sets gracefully, exquisitely, with his last exhale. He is free, he has let go. And I know that I must do the same.

ALZHEIMER'S IN THE FAMILY
ANN MARSHALL YOUNG

I remember as a child watching my paternal grandmother wordlessly cutting pictures out of magazines and saving them as precious valuables. Now, knowing she had the same Alzheimer's that later took my father, I am touched by her actions and see in them an appreciation of beauty, whatever the form, and a desire to save it from loss, just as so much else was slipping away from her.

I saw another side of Alzheimer's when my mother was ill with a recurrence of breast cancer. I realized at some point that Daddy couldn't really take care of her because he had some symptoms of dementia. Mama had hinted at problems in the preceding years, but it was only with her illness that I saw more clearly what was happening. Daddy was obviously not handling things well, either in his judgment or his emotional reactions. He was a retired physician, so should have been able to help with her care, but would argue that she did not need medical care and refuse to take her to her oncologist, as if this was a threat to his own self-esteem and medical knowledge.

As a result of all this, I spent much of the last several months of Mama's life with them, enabled to do so by being permitted in my job to work in the city where they lived. In spite of Daddy's issues, including hiding Mama's medicine and arguing with her doctors and nurses (some of whom could deal with his behavior better than others), I did my best to manage things and take care of her. He became angry with me for just being there, even hitting me once. Daddy had not been a great father to me, and we had had our clashes over the years, but this was far worse. I felt sympathy for him at times but also despair at how difficult he made things for Mama during her last months. She, who like so many spouses of those with Alzheimer's, ended up dying before him.

I tried to give Mama what I could, in spite of it all. It was heart-breaking to watch her waste away. As a beloved mother, grandmother, teacher, and community contributor, she had given, and meant, so much to so many. Then, when she died, I felt as if I'd lost a part of myself, and Daddy's continuing erratic behavior made that sorrow nearly unbearable. He would switch between fury, need, and denial.

I began going back and forth between home and checking on Daddy when I could. After a time, I discovered he had been sending blank checks through the mail to pay bills, and saw that he was losing the ability to write legibly. Then, his hometown banker called me with more concerns, about his coming in with "a woman" and taking out large amounts of cash. Since he didn't have unlimited funds, it was suggested I begin handling bills and money for him, as had been earlier directed by my mother and finalized in legal documents. Daddy also often got lost driving and had several accidents, until I finally had to "borrow" his car and "lose" his keys.

Then, at long last, I was able to get him to move to a facility where he would be more protected, when he discovered a woman he liked was living there. This was followed some time later by author-ities there telling me he needed a higher level of care, which led to his finally agreeing to come to a place in the city where my sister, a nurse, and I lived.

Having him where we were made things easier, especially with my sister helping. Ironically, as he became more compromised by the Alzheimer's, he also became calmer emotionally, at least with us. I did, however, sometimes have to address complaints about his behav-ior with others. His improvement with me was nice, even as I realized that he no longer knew who I was. He would sometimes treat me with ultimate courtesy, but on the other hand, at least once he made a physical "pass" at me—not having any idea, of course, that I was his daughter. Fortunately, I had been warned of this possibility by a psychologist I knew.

My sister and I learned a lot by attending support groups for families of Alzheimer's patients, where we could compare notes and share suggestions on how to deal with the difficulties and pain of it all. I had previously learned much, from a different perspective, of how Alzheimer's can affect families, when, as an administrative law judge, I had heard cases involving whether patients met certain state medical criteria for Medicaid to pay for their nursing home care. I had seen grown children of Alzheimer's patients break down crying when they shared their experiences of how the disease affected their parents, loved ones, and themselves, in so many ways.

I learned how parents with Alzheimer's will sometimes pit one adult child against another, charging that the main caregiver treats them poorly or unfairly, resulting in families harshly splitting up over the care of that parent. This knowledge helped me when Daddy railed against me trying to "take over" things that he wanted to do, leading my siblings to express feelings toward me ranging from doubt to hostility. Fortunately, over time, all of them came to see what was actually happening, but it was a tough time. I knew other families that never came together again, not understanding what I had been lucky enough to learn.

There were some occasions that helped our general outlook on things. Once, at a reunion of old neighbors where all our remaining family had gathered, Daddy spied an old friend from across a picnic table, who looked very much like our red-haired Mama. "Here's that sweet woman," he cried. "I've been looking everywhere for you!" We all beamed at this sign of his continuing love of our mama, despite all.

As time passed, Daddy lost more and more of himself, and soon he was hardly talking any sense at all. We gave him stuffed animals as gifts at this point, as he became more and more childlike. Daddy, who had been such a smart man, now reduced to this. To avert the sadness, we, his children and grandchildren, would play with him as with a child, laughing with him and some of the other patients as they engaged in their unique play.

Then he had a fall—often a precursor to the last decline. This led to his hospitalization, where my sister and I fed him until he was well enough to return to the nursing home. By this time, he was no longer talking at all. He also began to lose the ability to swallow, but the nurses would bring ice cream, which would just slide down his throat. He seemed to enjoy this, so I would sit with him and feed him ice cream.

The last time I did this, a few days before he died, at one point he seemed to look directly at me, as if there was some awareness of who I was. This may have been my imagination, but he seemed somehow to know it was me. And there appeared to be tears in his eyes. It was as if he wanted to tell me something.

Was this possible? Some months earlier, I had seen him flip from hallucinating and talking nonsense to being sharp as a tack for a quick moment, to address an overheard comment about himself. And I had heard him, within just the previous month or so, haltingly trying to count numbers, as if working against Alzheimer's by exercising his brain through somehow-remembered knowledge from his earlier medical career. And doing so with the pride of a child reciting his ABC's. Little bits and pieces of lucidity and humor in the midst of everything.

So I wondered whether it was possible he really was somehow trying to communicate with me. I don't actually know what was going on in what was left of his mind, but I hold on to that image of him looking at me and like to believe there was some consciousness there on his part, some desire to impart a message to me. And the message some part of me felt—or at least hoped was true—that last visit with him, was that he was asking my forgiveness for not having been a good father to me and telling me that he loved me.

I think of this from time to time, especially in those moments when I look into my own future and fear the day this disease may begin to take bits and pieces of me. And dearly hope some lovely lucid pieces remain.

STRANGER THAN
FICTION

INTRODUCTION

A fictional meditation on Alzheimer's and other dementias is a coat of many colors: tender, strong, curious, familiar, heartbreaking. And always a reflection of who we the readers are and who we could become. Fiction with dementia as part of the thematic tapestry is always about more than dementia. The stories are "about" the main character as somebody's somebody—mother, father, son, daughter, husband, friend. The funhouse mirror of fiction, both truly true and built on "make believe" through the winding road of the story, gives us back and unto ourselves as we inarguably are—indifferent and loyal, cowardly, misguided, terrified, and stubborn in the face of a disease that evokes a unique and chilling kind of terror.

Poetry springs from the soul. Fiction is rooted in the depths of our dreams and fears. Fiction walks the thin line between truth and emotion, fact and what if. It walks that line and crosses it again and again. Fiction is an open wound, a crooked smile, an unflinching gaze. Fiction reminds us that there is much we cannot escape, illness, affliction, pain, life itself, and the reality of redemption. How can there possibly be the right words, enough words, accurate words to describe and "recreate" the dementia-mind? Because there are right words, enough words, accurate words to describe and "recreate" all human horrors and human fears. Writers are blessed and cursed with a relentless insatiable will to know . . . everything and that will pick the lock on every mystery. An Alzheimer's story will always affirm that in the end there is no forgetting, there is only what we ache to remember and what we wish could forget. There is no forgetting, there is what we will take with us and what we will leave behind.

SUNRISE, SUNSET
EDWIDGE DANTICAT

1

It comes on again on her grandson's christening day. A lost moment, a blank spot, one that Carole does not know how to measure. She is there one second, then she is not. She knows exactly where she is, then she does not. Her older church friends tell similar stories about their surgeries, how they count backward from ten with an oxygen mask over their faces, then wake up before reaching one, only to find that hours, and sometimes even days, have gone by. She feels as though she were experiencing the same thing.

Her son-in-law, James, a dreadlocked high-school math teacher, is holding her grandson, Jude, who has inherited her daughter's globe-shaped head, penny-colored skin, and long fingers, which he wraps around Carole's chin whenever she holds him. Jude is a lively giggler. His whole body shakes when he laughs. Carole often stares at him for hours, hoping that his chubby face will bring back memories of her own children at that age, memories that are quickly slipping away.

Her daughter, Jeanne, is still about sixty pounds overweight on Jude's christening day, seven months after his birth. Jeanne is so miserable about this—and who knows what else—that she spends most days in her bedroom, hiding. Since her daughter is stuck in a state of mental fragility, Carole welcomes the opportunity to join Jude's other grandmother, Grace, in watching their grandson as often as she's asked. Carole likes to entertain Jude with whatever children's songs and peekaboo games she can still remember, including one she calls Solèy Leve, Solèy Kouche—Sunrise, Sunset—which she used to play with her children. She drapes a black sheet over her grandson's playpen and pronounces it "sunset," then takes the sheet off and calls it "sunrise." Her grandson does not seem to mind when she gets confused and reverses the order. He doesn't know the difference anyway.

Sometimes Carole forgets who Grace is and mistakes her for the nanny. She does, however, remember that Grace disapproved of her son's marrying Jeanne, whom she believed was beneath him. That censure now seems justified by Jeanne's failures as a mother.

Jeanne, Carole thinks, has never known real tragedy. Growing up in a country ruled by a merciless dictator, Carole watched her neighbors being dragged out of their houses by the dictator's denim-uniformed henchmen. One of her aunts was beaten almost to death for throwing herself in front of her husband as he was being arrested. Carole's father left the country for Cuba when she was twelve and never returned. Her mother's only means of survival was cleaning the houses of people who were barely able to pay her.

Carole's best friend lived next door, in another tin-roofed room, rented separately from the same landlord. During the night, while her mother slept, Carole often heard her friend being screamed at by her own mother, who seemed to hate her for being a burden. Carole tried so hard to protect her U.S.-born children from these stories that they are now incapable of overcoming any kind of sadness. Not so much her son, Paul, who is a minister, but Jeanne, whom she named after her childhood friend. Her daughter's psyche is so feeble that anything can rattle her. Doesn't she realize that the life she is living is an accident of fortune? Doesn't she know that she is an exception in this world, where it is normal to be unhappy, to be hungry, to work nonstop and earn next to nothing, and to suffer the whims of everything from tyrants to hurricanes and earthquakes?

The morning of her grandson's christening, Carole is wearing a long-sleeved white lace dress that she can't recall putting on. She has combed her hair back in a tight bun that now hurts a little. Earlier in the week, she watched from the terrace of her daughter's third-floor apartment as Jeanne dipped her feet in the condo's kidney-shaped communal pool. She'd walked out onto the terrace to look at the water, the unusual cobalt-blue color it becomes in late afternoon and the slow ripple of its surface, even when untouched by a breeze or bodies.

"I won't christen him!" Jeanne was shouting on the phone. "That's her thing, not ours."

"We're up soon," James says, snapping Carole out of her reverie. He is using the tone of voice with which he speaks to Jude. It's clear that this is not the first time he's told her this. Her daughter is looking neither at her nor at the congregation full of Carole's friends. She's not even looking at Jude, who has been dressed, most likely by James, in a plain white romper. Jeanne stares at the floor, as others take turns holding Jude and keeping him quiet in the church: first Grace, then Carole's husband, Victor, then James's younger sister, Zoe, who is the godmother, then James's best friend, Marcos, the godfather.

Carole keeps reminding herself that her daughter is still young. Only thirty-two. Jeanne was once a satisfied young woman, a guidance counselor at the school where James teaches. (When James and Jeanne first started dating, their friends called them J.J.; then Jude was born, and the three of them became Triple J.)

"She used to like children, right?" Carole sometimes asks Victor. "Before she had her son?"

When Jude's name is called from the pulpit by his uncle Paul, James motions for them to approach the altar. Paul, dressed in a long white ministerial robe, steps down from the pulpit and, while Jude is still in his father's arms, traces a cross on his forehead with scented oil. The oil bothers Jude's eyes and he wails. Undeterred, Paul takes Jude and begins praying so loudly that he shocks Jude into silence. After the prayer, he hands Jude back to his mother. Jeanne kisses her son's oil-soaked forehead and her eyes balloon with tears.

Carole knows that her daughter is not enjoying any of this, but she has found comfort in such rituals and she believes that her grandson will not be protected against the world's evils—including his mother's lack of interest in him—until this one is performed.

Later, at the post-christening lunch at her daughter's apartment, Carole spots James and Jeanne walking out of their bedroom. Jude is in Jeanne's arms. They have changed the boy out of his plain romper into an even plainer sleeveless onesie. Jeanne stops in the doorway and lowers a bib over Jude's face and murmurs, "Sunset." Then she raises the bib and squeals, "Sunrise!"

Watching her daughter play this game with the baby, Carole feels as though she herself were going through the motions, raising and lowering the bib. Not at this very moment but at some point in the hazy past. It's as if Jeanne had become Carole and James had become her once dapper and lanky husband, Victor, who now walks with a cane that he is always tapping against the ground.

All is not lost, Carole thinks. Her daughter has learned a few things from her, after all. Then it returns again, that all too familiar sensation of herself waning. What if she never recognizes anyone again? What if she forgets her husband? What if she stops remembering what it's like to love him, a feeling that has changed so much over the years, in ways that her daughter's love for her own husband seems also to be changing, even though James, like Victor, is patient. She's never seen him shout at or scold Jeanne. He doesn't even tell her to get out of bed or pay more attention to their child. He tells Carole and his own mother that Jeanne just needs time. But how long will this kind of tolerance last? How long can anyone bear to live with someone whose mind wanders off to a place where their love no longer exists?

Carole's husband is the only one who knows how far along she is. He is constantly subjected to her sudden mood changes, her bursts of anger followed by total stillness. He has tried for years to help her hide her symptoms, or lessen them with puzzles and other educational games, with coconut oil and omega-3 supplements, which she takes with special juices and teas. He is always turning off appliances, finding keys she's stored in unusual places like the oven or the freezer. He helps her finish sentences, nudges her to let her know if she has repeated something a few times. But maybe one day he will grow tired of this and put her in a home, where strangers will have to take care of her.

When Jude was born, Victor bought Carole a doll so that she could practice taking care of their grandson. It's a brown boy doll with a round face and tight peppercorn curls, like Jude's. When she puts the doll in the bath, its hair clings to its scalp, just like Jude's. Bathing the doll, then dressing it before bed, makes her feel calm, helps her sleep more soundly. But this, like her illness, is still a secret between her husband and her, a secret that they may not be able to keep much longer.

2

How do you become a good mother? Jeanne wants to ask someone, anyone. She wishes she'd been brave enough to ask her mother before her dementia, or whatever it is that she is suffering from, set in. Her mother refuses to have tests done and get a definitive diagnosis, and her father is fine with that.

"You don't poke around for something you don't want to find," he's told her a few times.

Her father offers the first toast at the christening lunch. "To Jude, who brought us together today," he says in Creole, then in English.

James hands Jeanne a champagne glass, which she has trouble balancing while holding their son. Her mother puts her own glass down and reaches over and takes Jude from Jeanne's arms.

"I'll toast with him," Carole says, and Jeanne fears her mother may actually believe that Jude's body is a champagne glass. She is afraid these days to let her mother hold her son, to leave them alone together, but since she and James are close by and Jude isn't fussing or fidgeting she does not protest.

After the toast, James asks if he can get Jeanne and her mother a plate of food. Carole nods, then quickly changes her mind. "Maybe later," she says. Jude is looking up at her now, his baby eyes fixed on her wrinkled and weary-looking face.

Carole isn't eating much these days. Jeanne, on the other hand, feels as though a deep and sour hole were burrowing through her body, an abyss that is always demanding to be filled.

Her husband doesn't insist. It's not his style. Throughout their courtship and marriage, he's never pressured her to do anything. Everything is always presented to her as a suggestion or a recommendation. It's as if he were constantly practicing being patient for the rowdy kids he teaches at school. Even there, he never loses his temper. Her mother, on the other hand, has been lashing out lately, though afterward she seems unable to remember doing it. She has always been a quiet woman. She is certainly kinder than James's mother, who wouldn't have given Jeanne or Carole the time of day if it weren't for James.

Jeanne often wonders if her mother was happier in Haiti. She doubts it. Jeanne has no right to be sad, her mother has often told her. Only Carole has the right to be sad, because she has seen and heard terrible things. Jeanne's father's approach to life is different. He is more interested than anybody Jeanne knows in the pleasure of joy, or the joy of pleasure, however you want to put it. It's as if he had sworn to enjoy every second of his life—to wear the best clothes he can afford, to eat the best food, to go to dances where his favorite Haitian bands are playing.

Victor drove a city bus for most of Jeanne's childhood, then when he got older he switched to driving a taxicab. Between fares, he sat in the parking lot at Miami International Airport, discussing Haitian politics with his cabdriver friends. Perhaps her mother wouldn't be losing her mind if she'd worked outside their home. Church committees and family were her life's work, a luxury they'd been able to afford because Victor worked double shifts and took extra weekend jobs. Carole could have worked, if she'd wanted to, as a lunch lady in a school cafeteria or as an elder companion or a nanny, like many of her church friends.

Jeanne never wanted to be a housewife like her mother, but here she is now, stuck at home with her son. She doesn't leave the house much anymore, except for her son's doctor's appointments. Most of the time, she's afraid to leave her bed, afraid even to hold her son, for fear that she might drop him or hug him too tightly and smother him. Then the fatigue sets in, an exhaustion so forceful it doesn't even allow her to sleep. Motherhood is a kind of foggy bubble she can't step out of long enough to wrap her arms around her child.

Oddly enough, he's an easy child. He's been sleeping through the night since the day they brought him home. He naps regularly. He isn't colicky or difficult. He is just there.

James decides to offer a toast of his own. He taps his champagne glass with a spoon to catch everyone's attention.

"I want to make a toast to my wife, not only for being a phenomenal wife and mother but for bravely bringing Jude into our lives," he says.

Why does he want to think of her as brave? Perhaps he's thinking of the twenty-six hours of labor that ended in a C-section, during which her son was pulled out with the umbilical cord wrapped around his neck. He had nearly died, the doctor told her, because of her stubborn insistence on a natural birth.

The pregnancy had been easy. She'd worked a regular schedule until the day she went into labor. The pain was intense, pulsating, throbbing, but bearable, even after the twenty-fifth hour. First babies can put you through the wringer, the nurses kept telling her, but the second one will be easier.

She was lucky, blessed, her mother said, that the baby was saved in time.

After his toast, her husband kisses her cheek.

"Hear, hear," her brother says in his booming minister's voice.

Jeanne's eyes meet her husband's and she wishes that a new spark would pass between them, something to connect them still, besides their child. She feels like crying, but she does not want to incite one of her mother's rants about her being a spoiled brat who needs to stop sulking and get on with her life. In all the time since her child was born and she realized that his birth would not necessarily make her joyful, and in all the time since she became aware that her mother's mind, as well as her mother's love, was slipping away, today at the church was the first time she has cried.

3

A week before Jude was born, Carole went to the Opa Locka Hialeah Flea Market, which Haitians called Ti Mache, and got some eucalyptus leaves and sour oranges for her daughter's first postpartum bath. She bought her daughter a corset and a few yards of white muslin, which she sewed into a bando for Jeanne to wrap around her belly. But because of the C-section neither the bath nor the binding was possible, which was why her daughter's belly did not go back to the way it had been before. Jeanne became larger, in fact, because she refused to drink the fennel and aniseed infusions that both Carole and Grace brewed for her. And she refused to breastfeed, which would not only have melted her extra fat but would also have made her feel less sad.

When Jeanne and Paul were babies, no other woman was around to help. Carole didn't have the luxury of lying in bed while relatives took care of her and her children. Her husband did the best he could. He went out and got her the leaves and made her the teas. He gave her the baths himself. He helped her retie the bando every morning before he left for work, but during the hours that he was gone she was so lonely and homesick that she kept kissing her babies' faces, as if their cheeks were plots of land in the country she'd left behind.

She couldn't imagine life without her children. She would have felt even more lost and purposeless without them. She wanted them both to have everything they desired. And whenever money was tight, especially after she and Victor bought their house in Miami's Little Haiti, she would clean other people's homes while her children were at school and her husband was at work, something her husband never knew about. Her secret income made him admire her even more. Every week, before he handed her the allowance for household expenses, he would proudly tell the children, "Your manman sure knows how to stretch a dollar."

Her cleaning money also paid for all the things her daughter believed she'd be a pariah without—brand-name sneakers and clothes, class rings, prom dresses. Her son wasn't interested in anything but books, and only library books at that. He would happily walk around with holes in his cheap shoes.

She should have told her daughter about the sacrifices she'd made. If she had, it would be easier now to tell her that she couldn't stay sad forever. Where would the family be if Carole had stayed sad when she arrived in this country? Sometimes you just have to shake the devil off you, whatever that devil is. Even if you don't feel like living for yourself, you have to start living for your child, for your children.

4

Jeanne doesn't realize that her husband and her mother have wandered off with Jude until she finds herself alone with her father.

She hasn't discussed her mother's condition with him for some time. She does not want to tell him or her husband how earlier in the week, when her mother was visiting, she'd forced herself to go out and sit by the pool while her son was napping. As soon as she put her feet in the water, she glanced up and saw her mother watching her from the terrace. Her mother looked bewildered, as though she had no idea where she was. Jeanne was in the middle of a phone call with James. She ended the call quickly and ran upstairs, and by the time she reached the apartment her mother was standing by the door. She pushed the door shut, grabbed Jeanne by the shoulders, and slammed her into it. Had Carole been bigger, she might have cracked open Jeanne's head.

Jeanne kept saying, "Mommy, Mommy," like an incantation, until it brought her back.

"What happened?" her mother asked.

Jeanne wanted to call an ambulance, or at least her father, but she was in shock and her mother seemed fine the rest of the day. Jeanne avoided her as much as she could, let her watch a talk show she liked, and made sure that she was not left alone with Jude.

The next day, her mother showed up after James had gone to work and began shouting at her in Creole. "You have to fight the devil," she yelled. "Stop being selfish and living for yourself. Start living for your child."

Those incidents have made Jeanne afraid both of and for her mother. She agreed to go through with the christening in the hope that it might help. Maybe her mother was only pretending to be losing her mind in order to get her way.

Sitting next to James on their living room sofa, with Jude in her arms, Carole appears calmer than she has all week. Paul is sitting on the other side of her, and the three of them seem to be talking about Jude, or about children in general. Then James's friend Marcos joins them, and Jude reaches out for his big cloud of an Afro.

Jeanne wonders how her brother could fail to notice that their mother is deteriorating. In all their conversations about the christening, he never mentioned Carole's state of mind. Was it because he was used to seeing her as a pious woman, not as his mother but as his "sister" in the Lord? Paul has never paid much attention to practical things. He spent most of their childhood reading books that even the adults they knew had never heard of, obscure novels and anthropological studies, the biographies of famous theologians and saints. Before he officially joined their mother's church, when he was a senior in high school, he had considered becoming a priest. He was always more concerned about the next world than he was about this one.

Her mother motions for Paul to scoot over, then lowers Jude into the space between them on the sofa. Jude turns his face back and forth and keeps looking up at the adults, especially at James.

"How are you these days?" Jeanne's father asks. As he speaks to Jeanne, he's looking at her mother in a way she has never seen before, with neither admiration nor love but alarm, or even distress.

"OK," she says. Usually that is enough for him. Her father, like her husband, doesn't usually push. But this time he does.

"Why do all this today?" her father asks, though he already knows the answer. "Did you have this child for her, too? Because she won't be able to take care of him for you. You'll have to do it for yourself."

"Of course I didn't have my son for her," Jeanne says.

"Then why have him?" he asks. "It doesn't seem like you want him."

This, whatever it is that she is feeling, she wants to tell him, isn't about not wanting her son. It's about not being up to the task; the job is too grand, too permanent, even with her husband's help. It's hard to explain to her father or to anyone else, but something that was supposed to kick in, maybe a light that was meant to turn on in her head, never did. Despite her complete physical transformation, at times she feels as though she had not given birth at all. It's not that she doesn't want her son, or wishes he hadn't been born; it's just that she can't believe that he is truly hers.

She's desperate to change the subject.

"What's really wrong with Manman?" she asks.

"We're not done talking about you," her father says.

"What's wrong with her?" she insists.

"She's not herself," he says.

"It's more than that."

"What do you want me to say?"

"We need to know the truth."

"We," he says, pointing to her mother, then to himself, "already know the truth."

Jeanne hears her mother laughing, softly at first then louder, at something that either James or Marcos has said. She realizes that possibly there have been doctors, a diagnosis, one that her parents are keeping to themselves.

"What are you saying?" she asks.

"I'll soon have to put her somewhere," he says.

She thinks of the expense and how her mother will not be the only one who is dislocated. Her father may have to sell the house in order to afford a decent place where her mother won't be neglected or abused. She thinks of the irony of her family's not being able to take care of her mother, who has dedicated so much of her life to them.

"I'm not saying it will happen tomorrow, but we'll have to put her somewhere one day."

Jeanne hasn't seen the pain in her father's face before, because she hasn't been looking for it. She hasn't been thinking about other people's pain at all. But now she can see the change in him. His hair is grayer and his voice drags. His eyes are red from lack of sleep, his face weathered with worry.

5

Carole and her childhood friend Jeanne used to talk to each other through a hole they'd poked in the plywood that separated their rooms. In the morning, when Jeanne went to fetch water at the neighborhood tap, she would whistle a wake-up call to Carole. Jeanne's whistle sounded like the squeaky chirping of a pipirit gri, the gray kingbirds that flew around the area until boys knocked them down with slingshots, roasted them in fire pits, and ate them.

One morning, Jeanne did not whistle, and Carole never saw her again. The boys in the neighborhood said that her mother had killed her and buried her, then disappeared, but Jeanne's mother had probably just been unable to make the rent and skipped out before daylight.

The next occupant of that room was Victor. Victor's father worked on a ship that often traveled to Miami, and everyone in the neighborhood knew that Victor would be going there, too, one day. His father brought back suitcases full of clothes a couple of times a year, and Victor would always come over with some T-shirts or dresses that his mother said she had no use for. Victor soon discovered the hole in the plywood and would slip his finger through and wave it at her. Then she would whistle to him, like the last kingbird of their neighborhood.

Carole knew from the moment she met Victor that he would take care of her. She never thought he'd conspire against her, or even threaten to put her away. But here he is now, plotting against her with a woman she does not know, a fleshy, pretty woman, just the way he once liked them, just the way she was, when he liked her most.

Her husband and this woman are speaking in whispers. What are they talking about? And why is she sitting next to this peppercorn-haired doll that her husband sometimes uses to trick her, pretending it's a real baby. Her real babies are gone. They disappeared with her friend Jeanne, and all she has left is this doll her husband bought her.

She looks around the room to see if anyone else can see what's going on, how this young woman is trying to steal her husband from her right under her nose, while she is stuck on this sofa between strangers and a propped-up baby doll. She grabs the doll by its armpits and raises it to her shoulder. The doll's facial expressions are so real, so lifelike, that its lips curl and its cheeks crumple as though it were actually about to cry. To calm it down, she whistles the pipit's spirited squeak.

Carole is trying to explain all this to the men on either side of her, but they can't understand her. One of them holds his hands out to her as if he wanted her to return the doll to him.

They are crowding around her now. The fleshy young woman, too, is moving closer. Carole doesn't understand what all the fuss is about. She just wants to take the doll out to the yard, the way she often does when her husband isn't around. She wants to feel the sun-filled breeze on her face and see the midday luster of the pool. She wants to prove to everyone that not only can she take care of herself but she can take care of this doll, too.

6

How does her mother get past James and Paul and run to the terrace with Jude in her arms? Jude is squirming and wailing, his bare pudgy legs cycling erratically as her mother dangles him over the terrace railing.

Her father is the first to reach the terrace, followed by James and everyone else. Though Carole is standing on the shady side of the terrace, she is sweating. Her bun has loosened as though Jude, or someone else, had been pulling at it.

Jeanne isn't sure how long her mother's bony arms will be able to support her son, especially since Jude is crying and twisting, all while turning his head toward the faces on the terrace as though he knew how desperate they were to have him back inside.

Paul has rushed downstairs, and Jeanne is now looking down at his face as she tries to figure out where her son might land if her mother drops him. The possibility of his landing in Paul's arms is as slim or as great as his landing in the pool or on the ficus hedge below the terrace.

Marcos also appears down by the pool, as does James's sister, Zoe, adding more hands for a possible rescue. James is on the phone with the police. Grace has Jeanne caged in her arms, as if to keep her from crumbling to the floor. Her father is standing a few feet from her mother, begging, pleading.

Once James is off the phone, he switches places with her father. Jude balls his small fists, reopens them, then aims both his hands at his father. He stops crying for a moment, as if waiting for James to grab him. When James reaches for him, Carole pushes him farther out. Everyone gasps and, once Grace releases Jeanne, she doubles over, as if she had been sliced in two.

"Mommy, please," Jeanne says, straightening herself up. "Souple Manman. Tanpri Manman."

Other tenants come out of their apartments. Some are already on their terraces. Others are by the pool with Paul, Zoe, and Marcos. Her son at his last checkup weighed twenty-seven pounds, which is about a fifth of her mother's current weight. Her mother will not be able to hold on to him much longer.

Jeanne walks toward her husband, approaching carefully, brushing past her father, who appears to be in shock.

"Manman, please give me my baby," Jeanne says. She tries to speak in a firm and steady voice, one that will not frighten her son.

Her mother regards her with the dazed look that is now too familiar.

"Let me have him, Carole," Jeanne says. Maybe not being her daughter will give her more authority in her mother's eyes. Her mother may think that Jeanne is someone she has to listen to, someone she must obey.

"Baby," her mother says, and it sounds more like a term of endearment for Jeanne than like the realization that she's holding a small child.

"Your baby?" Carole asks, her arms wavering now, as if she were finally feeling Jude's full weight.

Jeanne lowers her voice. "He's my child, Manman. Please give him to me."

Jeanne can see in the loosening of her mother's arms that she is returning. But her mother is still not fully back, and, if she returns too suddenly, she may get confused and drop Jude. While her mother's eyes are focused on her, she signals with a nod for her husband to move in, and, with one synchronized lurch, her father reaches for her mother and her husband grabs their son. Her mother relaxes her grip on Jude only after he is safely back across the railing.

James collapses on the terrace floor, his still crying son pressed tightly against his chest. Jeanne's father takes her mother by the hand and leads her back inside. He sits with her on the sofa and wraps his arms around her as she calmly rests her head on his shoulder.

Two police officers, two black women, arrive soon after. They are followed by EMTs. A light is shined in her mother's pupils by one of the EMTs, then her blood pressure is taken. Though her mother seems to have snapped out of her episode and now only looks tired, it's determined that Carole needs psychiatric evaluation. Jude is examined and has only some bruising under his armpits from his grandmother's tight grip.

Jeanne sees the dazed look return to her mother's eyes as she climbs onto the lowered gurney, with some help from Victor and from Paul. Her father asks that her mother not be strapped down, but the head EMT insists that it is procedure and promises not to hurt her.

Jeanne had hoped that her mother was only trying to teach her a lesson, to shock her out of her blues and remind her that she is capable of loving her son, but then she sees her mother's eyes as she is being strapped to the gurney. They are bleary and empty. She seems to be looking at Jeanne but is actually looking past her, at the wall, then at the ceiling.

Carole's body goes limp as the straps are snapped over her wrists and ankles, and it seems as though she were letting go completely, giving in to whatever has been ailing her. She seems to know that she'll never be back here, at least not in the way she was before. She seems to know, too, that this moment, unlike a birth, is no new beginning.

7

Carole wished she'd see more of this, her daughter and her son-in-law together with their baby boy. James's arms are wrapped around his wife, as she holds their son, who has fallen asleep. Perhaps Jeanne will now realize how indispensable her son is to her. Carole regrets not telling her daughter a few of her stories. Now she will never get to tell them to her grandson, either. She will never play with him again.

The first time her husband took her to the doctor, before all the brain scans and spinal taps, the doctor asked about her family's medical history. He asked whether her parents or her grandparents had suffered from any mental illnesses, Alzheimer's, or dementia. She had not been able to answer any of his questions, because when he asked she could not remember anything about herself.

"She's not a good historian," the doctor told her husband, which was, according to Victor, the doctor's way of saying that she was incapable of telling her own life story.

She is not a good historian. She never has been. Even when she was well. Now she will never get a chance to be. Her grandson will grow up not knowing her. The single most memorable story that will exist about her and him will be of her dangling him off a terrace, in what some might see as an attempt to kill him. For her, all this will soon evaporate, fade away. But everyone else will remember.

They are about to roll her out of the apartment on the gurney. Although her wrists are strapped down, her son is holding her left hand tightly. Jeanne gives Jude to his other grandmother and walks over to the gurney. She moves her face so close to Carole's that Carole thinks she is going to bite her. But then Jeanne pulls back and it occurs to Carole that she is playing Alo, Bye, another peekaboo game her children used to enjoy. With their faces nearly touching, Jeanne crinkles her nose and whispers, "Alo, Manman," then "Bye, Manman."

It would be appropriate, if only she could make herself believe that this is what her daughter is actually doing. It would be a fitting close to her family life, or at least to life with her children. You are always saying hello to them while preparing them to say goodbye to you. You are always dreading the separations, while cheering them on, to get bigger, smarter, to crawl, babble, walk, speak, to have birthdays that you hope you'll live to see, that you pray they'll live to see. Jeanne will now know what it's like to live that way, to have a part of yourself walking around unattached to you, and to love that part so much that you sometimes feel as though you were losing your mind.

Her daughter reaches down and takes her right hand, so that both of her children are now holding her scrawny, shaky hands, which seem not to belong to her at all.

"Mèsi Manman," her daughter says. "Thank you."

There is nothing to thank her for. She has only done her job, her duty as a parent. There is no longer any need for hellos or goodbyes, either. Soon there will be nothing left, no past to cling to, no future to hope for. Only now.

THE BEACHES OF HAZEL SASSO
HEATHER L. DAVIS

A warm mist curled up the Amalfi coast, turning the dark to velvet. No place was so beautiful to Hazel Sasso, and in no place had she been so alone. While the children slept, she walked, even though her mother-in-law said the whole town would gossip. No happy wife walks the cliffs at midnight. But Joe, her husband, was out at sea. She could spend hours staring at the waves as they crashed below, wondering when she would feel his arms around her again.

She sat down at the cliff's edge and sang *Joseph Sasso* to herself, his name both a riddle and a curse as she looked down at the rocky shore. Sometimes she wondered if she loved him too much, or if he loved the sea more than her loved her. But then she begged forgiveness in her mind. He was a wonderful husband and father, when he was there. And she had finally learned the ways of the small Italian town near the naval base where he'd been stationed. Nothing happened quickly here, and no one was ever on time. She'd had to let go of American impatience.

As a girl, she'd dreamed of leaving South Jersey but never imagined she'd live near Naples, Italy, married to a wise-cracking Italian-American sailor. He promised someday they'd all move back to the States. He'd finish with the Navy and open a deli. She could be with her family, bake fancy wedding and birthday cakes to sell.

The briny salt breeze settled on her tongue. Or maybe it was the saltiness of a tear. It surprised her because she did not have the time or space to cry—she had too much to do and was no helpless victim. She'd set up and was running a household in a foreign country practically by herself. She had gotten the kids settled in school and was learning a new language. As she wiped her eyes, a little angry at herself, she saw a tall dark-haired figure to her right, a man far below, close to the water. She wanted to know who he was—he seemed familiar. She stood up and tried to run toward him, but her legs wouldn't move the way she wanted them to.

By the time she reached the water, he was gone and the beach looked different, not like Italy at all. Where was she? Why couldn't she recognize this place? The contours of the land had changed. Panic stirred in her gut like a living creature, but she tamped it down. There were only three places she could be, the coast of Italy, New Jersey, or Delaware—the only coasts and beaches she had ever been too. It would come to her. It had to.

Hazel tried to shake off her slippers, but they wouldn't budge. So she sat and pulled them off, then stood up again slowly, feeling dizzy. She wanted the cold water on her feet.

Behind her a voice. Her mother's.

"Hazel, what in tarnation? Put those shoes back on."

"But Mama, please. I just want to dip my feet. I won't get my dress wet."

"That's what you say every time, Hazel. We have church in thirty minutes."

"Okay, I'm coming."

She dipped her feet anyway, even though the water seemed too cold now. Her mother never cared if her brothers got a little sandy or wet. They got away with everything, especially at Ocean City.

She backed up and almost toppled over. After looking for her shoes for a moment, she gave up and decided to stay barefoot. There was a boy down in Rehoboth she'd been hoping to see again someday. Maybe she could walk all the way there. She'd met him at a church camp sing-along. She'd dropped her hymnal, and he picked it up and handed it to her. His impersonation of the stiff and serious music director made her laugh. Later, on the beach not far from Dolle's Salt Water Taffy, they talked until her mother came looking for her, angrier than Hazel had ever seen her. The boy, Wendell, wrote her a letter a few weeks later. It wasn't a love letter, but it made her feel special. She kept it under her pillow. Only one person knew about it—her best friend, Sarah.

That looked like her farther down, toward the pier. It took Hazel a while, tromping through the sand, to reach the tall, gangly girl with red hair and a beautiful smile. They hugged tightly then plopped down in the damp sand.

Sarah was beside herself.

"You won't believe it, Haze."

"What? You look like you just got picked to be Miss America."

"It's better than that. Johnny Douglas just kissed me!"

"What? How did that happen?" Hazel felt giddy and strange.

"We went to the very end of the boardwalk where there was nobody around. We held hands. Then he did it."

"A real kiss?"

Sarah nodded violently. "A French kiss!"

Hazel marveled at this. She thought she was pretty enough with her wavy brown hair and blue eyes—though she was a little plump— but Wendell had only held her hand, not tried to kiss her. Maybe they ran out of time, or maybe she was too shy and quiet. Sarah was the opposite—bold and funny. That's probably why they were such good friends.

"I'll be back," Sarah said, popping up and brushing the sand from her butt. "Johnny's calling me."

Hazel watched her best friend spring across the dunes, the white polka dots on Sarah's blue one-piece bouncing away, getting smaller and smaller. "Give Johnny a kiss for me," Hazel called into the rising wind.

When had it gotten so blustery? Hazel didn't like the roughness of the waves or the way those fast-moving clouds blocked the moon. Henry might catch a chill. He loved storms and would not want to go into the beach house, but this was more than a little squall.

Hazel struggled to her feet, shivering. "Henry," she squeaked into the wind, her voice barely a whisper. His metal pail and shovel jutted from the sand.

Then she saw them—small footprints heading to the boardwalk. "That rascal."

At five years old, Henry had the determination of his namesake, Henry Ford. If he wanted something, almost nothing or no one could stop him. Distraction and relocation were the only ways Hazel could keep him in line—distracting him with something more exciting, at least for a few moments, or moving him to another place entirely.

He must have slipped away while she was arranging their blanket. She tried not to overreact. He couldn't be far. She started walking, looking as far as possible in every direction. Closer to the water, a couple were kissing passionately. Hazel squinted. It looked like two women—they were practically in each other's laps. Her mother and father would be shocked by this, but Hazel felt indifferent. Maybe they thought no one would notice them this late at night. She'd seen friends of friends beaten by their husbands and neighbors so lonely they took their own lives. How could any kind of real love be wrong? Live and let live, Hazel thought.

She wanted to ask them if they'd seen Henry but couldn't bring herself to interrupt. The footsteps went in the opposite direction anyway.

She walked left, then right, then left again. She was sure there had been a boardwalk here. Her heart beat faster as she imagined her only son running into the street and being hit by a car or picked up by a kidnapper. Or he might slip into the surf further down. She wrung her hands and called his name again and again.

The words sounded like marbles tumbling in the tide, making no sense.

Raindrops hit her shoulders and arms and head. She was tired of Joe being gone, of being both mother and father. She did want to cry sometimes, she had to admit. Maybe she should leave him and go back to the States. She was still young enough to find another husband.

Someone touched her shoulder from behind. She turned around.

"Joe?" Her heart almost stopped.

"Baby, I missed you so much," he said, cupping her cheek in his hand.

She couldn't believe he was finally home. He looked tired but more handsome than ever, his dark eyes pretty under thick lashes, that sly grin on his face.

"Don't leave me again," Hazel said and kissed him hard, like a movie star.

He smelled like starched cotton and lemon shaving cream, like sunburned skin and the sea. He was hers. Tears rolled down her cheeks as he wrapped his arms around her.

There was so much she wanted to tell Joe, so many days to describe—all the amazing things the kids had done, all the struggles big and small she'd had to overcome, how sometimes she couldn't sleep at all.

But the words wouldn't form. And now he was walking away. Grief rushed at her like a hurricane.

"Where are you going?"

"Gotta get my bags. Be right back."

"Okay," she said, letting out a sigh. He wasn't going back to the ship just yet.

But something wasn't right. Hazel felt exhausted, like she'd been running up a mountain. She wanted to wait for Joe but also wanted nothing more than to be home in her bed with the kids tucked in and Nonna drinking her nighttime tumbler of Chianti.

"Joe," she crooned in a voice like old floorboards. "Joe, Joe, Joe."

She could hear the ocean roaring behind her and the buzzing of lights on the boardwalk. She couldn't walk much farther or stand much longer. Maybe it was time to be done. She was curious though: Which country was this? What shore? Why couldn't she tell?

As Hazel frowned and started to shiver, a sharp brightness swept the sand. She covered her eyes. Someone was coming—a pack of them in dark clothes, maybe with guns. They were going to kill her. "Hazel!" they called. "Hazel Sasso!"

Hazel turned and tried to run. The sand kept pulling at her heels, making her sink. The wind ripped at her face. She wasn't ready to be captured, jailed, penned up. They were going to put her in a straitjacket and bolt every door. She'd read about this.

"Mama," said a voice. Someone ran toward her.

"Joe, help me!" she yelled. "Help!"

As she tried to run, she felt the earth tilt. Then they reached her, and a man started wrapping something big and soft around her. Too many people. They were rushing, trying to bring her down—policemen and policewomen with shiny badges and flashlights.

"Mama," the man said, touching her hair. "It's me—Henry. Your son. Thank God, we found you!"

She looked at his face. A little familiar but no, she didn't know this person. "You're not my son."

He wrapped the blanket tighter around her then took her face in his hands. "Mama, we were so worried. You're safe now. We've been looking for you for hours."

She shook her head, wrung her hands. "No, no, no, no."

The man who said he was Henry looked into her eyes. He had a kind face framed by wild brown hair, graying at the temples. His blue eyes were red and tired-looking. "Your name is Hazel Sasso. You have two children: me and a daughter named Sonia. She lives in Sea Isle City, New Jersey. You live in Rehoboth Beach with me. We're in Rehoboth Beach now. You have three grandchildren—Franny, Sarah, and Joe."

Hazel shook her head back and forth, back and forth.

"Mama, it's okay." He stroked her shoulder. "You're safe now. These nice people are helping us, and we need to get you dry. Do you understand? Should I sing Dad's favorite song?"

The young man covered Hazel's frigid hands with his warmer ones and started to hum. She couldn't help but listen. The tune was bouncy and bright. Something scratched at the outside of her mind like a cat at the basement door, desperate to get in. Henry had a long-haired Persian cat. He loved that cat. This man beside her had the most determined look on his face as he hummed, just like her son when he went looking for that cat.

"Henry?" she said, her gaze fully focused on him for the first time since the group had approached.

"Yes, yes. It's me." Henry smiled and exhaled, then nodded to the policeman and woman. "Let's get her to the car. She's soaking wet. Thank you so much for your help."

"Toast," she said. "With jam. I want toast. Do you have toast?"

"Of course. I'll make you toast—don't worry. Do you know where you are now?"

She nodded, calmer, steadier. She was Hazel Sasso, and this was her son, Henry. She had only wanted to go for a walk. He was a good boy, but he had grown up so quickly.

"Where are we, Mama?"

She swiveled her head weakly, gazing at the water, sky, and sand as if she'd never seen them before. "The beach, at night, in the rain."

"That's right. Which one, Mama? Which beach?"

She squeezed his hand and tried to remember. She wanted to tell him, but the name wouldn't come. What did it matter? Henry had found her and she'd seen Joe and Sarah, even though they left this world long ago. Sometimes she could remember events forty years in the past like they just happened but could not remember her own name.

Her brokenness made her furious, but there was nothing she could do. She stepped in the direction of the surf.

"Where are you going, Mama?" Henry said.

"Joe's coming back soon. I want to meet him."

Henry turned to the officers beside him. "I'm sorry. Just one minute."

He stepped toward the sea with his mother, his arms around her like she might melt away in the rain. "Mama, I'm here for you, but Dad is gone. He loved you very much. We all do."

Hazel kept her gaze on the mysterious black water until she felt it, that odd sensation, a feeling of something infinite, going on and on and on. Though it was wider and stronger than her, it was also inside of her, no matter how confused she became. She could not explain it with words because it held everything and everyone she'd ever loved.

"Mama," Henry said softly. "Are you okay?"

Hazel nodded slowly, her eyes never leaving the wild waves. "Yes, yes, yes," she half-sang to herself. "We're at the beach."

NEW WORLD
JULIE LANGSDORF

A new Cadillac every year from the rock-and-roll star son, the one who sends her three dozen roses on Valentine's Day, addressed "to my best girl."

Another son whose hands shake, who taps in the wrong number in his cell phone over and over, his face red enough to burst. "Monday we're putting you in a home, Ma. We're taking everything out of here and putting you in a home."

She answers with a laugh that makes her teeter on her high heels, makes her sugar-strand hair shiver on her bony head. Everything is white and breakable here, porcelain figurines, tea cups, narrow-stemmed lamps. There are wires and blinking lights everywhere, like a booby trap. If she falls, she'll shatter.

"Ma? Why you got so much crap in here?"

The third son calls her every day to tell her he's going to buy, then to sell, to buy and sell and buy and sell and buy and sell. "How are the kids?" she asks.

"Fine," he says. "They're a bunch of shitheads. They're fine."

She can't tell her sons apart any more. Not on the phone. Not in person. There are too many grandkids to count. Great-grandkids. Half grands and half greats. Step grandkids. Adopted kids. Ex-wives and second wives. Third-fourth-fifth wives. Mexican gardeners. Mexican cooks. Mexican nannies. She never learned Spanish. She never even learned English good.

She has a needlepoint framed on the wall of her kitchen. "Cooking sucks." A gift.

She's sitting in the little synagogue, her father praying out of tune, her little sister, the one who died, on her lap. She's walking on Rodeo Drive past dogs in shiny booties and cashmere coats. Chandeliers dangle from the lampposts. The leather jackets are velvet soft here, with no memory of where they came from. Her father was a cattle dealer. They used to keep the cows out back. Her sons don't want to know.

He drives like a nut, up and down the palm tree–studded hills, past the house with the statues where Rock Hudson lived, past Hugh Hefner's mansion. They had some good times there, by God. "Beautiful broads."

"What, Ma?"

"Nothing."

"You're out of your head, you old bat."

She laughs. Is she? Is she out of her head?

Barbara Streisand lives there. Larry King lives there. Frau Mueller lives on the corner. Herr Kunstler, the butcher, down the road. His son said he'd drown her if he caught her near the river. Martin told her to leave her window open at night. He threw in loaves of bread, *without which we would have starved.*

Dinner at a restaurant that's so dark you can't see the food. The waiter glides over with the bill like a man on ice skates.

"Let me see it."

"I'm paying, Ma."

She grabs it when he looks away. $3,465 for six people. Six bottles of wine at $400 each. "It tasted like cheap wine to me."

"That's because you're a peasant. You got peasant tastes."

"You're right!"

She dreamt she went back last night and knocked on doors to see who was still there. Martin answered. He was still twenty. *"Du lebst noch?"* he asked her. *You're still alive?*

The daughter-in-law sends her roasted chickens from a fancy shop. Every week, another chicken knocking at her door. "Why she spend all that money? I don't even like chicken." Should she freeze the stuffed peppers? She can't eat all this. She calls a son to see if he wants it. He tells her to shove it up her ass. "See you later, you bull-shitter," she says, laughing.

"Hi, you old bag." It's the rock star son, inviting her for Christmas, thirty people, four turkeys, catered on the beach. "I'll send a car for you."

She started going to temple again recently. It feels good. She doesn't eat pork. On Fridays.

Her sister is visiting from Palm Beach. They go to the Grove, to sit in the sunshine and watch people shop. They drink Caffé Americano, the cheapest thing on the menu. *They're meshuga, charging four dollars for a coffee, am I right?* Nights, they eat white fish salad and chopped liver and bagels and watch videos of the rock star son in concert. She doesn't like the music. You call that music?

"Ma, videos are shit." One of the sons says. "Throw out your videos, okay? And your records, too, while you're at it. And all that other crap you got in there. You got so much crap."

And yet they keep buying her more crap.

"Oh, my God, get a towel," she tells her sister. She's just had diarrhea on the couch. It was the sausage at lunch. Too spicy. "Don't use soap, only water," she says, the shit dripping down her leg. But her sister is gone, back in Palm Beach.

They say they're going to put her away. Do they mean it? She's afraid to ask.

She was a wild one. She loved the boys. Her father used to beat her every day. "And I deserved it." She was quite a dancer.

"You're out of your head, Ma."

"I used to dance all the time, and then one night at *Zum Lamm,* nobody would dance with me. *Dirty Jew*, they said. It broke my heart." She had an aunt in America. They got nearly everyone in the family out. Not the father. Not three of the sisters.

Her sons don't want to know.

"Why you got so much crap in here, Ma?"

If it were up to her, she'd keep three things. A button from her father's nightshirt. The pincushion her friend Idl gave her before the ship left for America. Idl had tears in her eyes. *Now we have no one.*

The photo of her family on her fifteenth birthday, in the meadow by the river, where they used to lay out their bedclothes to dry. They kept the smell of the outdoors on them when they brought them back inside. She used to smell hay and sunshine all night long, in her bed.

That's the thing, the one thing she'd keep. Just that. The smell of a sunny day in Gundelsheim, a sunny day before the world shattered.

CHARLEMAGNE
JOE A. OPPENHEIMER

Since forever, Dad was the first one up. Long before he had to show up at Rossetti's Auto Body, he'd brew himself the day's first espresso. Then he'd grab the paper from the yard, sit on the old plaid sofa, and watch the sunrise. Of course, he'd also be petting Charlie. After that ritual was completed and before the sun would be full up over the neighbor's roof, he'd stand, stretch, and put Charlie on a leash. By then other early risers would be up, walking their dogs.

Charlie would do his business and get his first social hour of the day. He was always more ready to socialize than Dad was. Dad never knew the names of our neighbors—even Mrs. Polakoff, who lived just two doors down and walked a fancy bichon frise that she was always having to clean. Charlie, on the other hand, knew all his neighbors, maybe not by name, but he sure was up close and personal with them. He'd tug at the leash furiously when he'd see the McDaniels's dachshund who, if I remember right, was called Schnitzel.

Charlie was a handsome and tall golden. His coat's sheen and his proud, youthful posture was a contrast to his master's slouch and demeanor. The picture caused many a passerby to steal a second glance of my father's stocky, dark, Central-European frame. Some say goldens are the friendliest (and dumbest) of all the breeds. Charlie sure was friendly. I don't think he ever had an enemy in the world. But I never thought he was dumb.

Most days they'd be gone pretty much a full hour. You couldn't miss their return. What with Charlie's happy barking, and my father's loud "Good fella, there, good boy!" he could have woken up

Grandfather, who was lying two miles away and six feet under. We'd all be up, and Mom would have breakfast started.

Dad was a welder at Rossetti's. They gave him a steady income and his addiction to espresso. If he'd been more sociable, he might have used the bragging rights he earned by working only a few miles from home in a town full of commuters. He could leave at a respectable hour and come home pretty early most evenings. Of course, when home, he'd grab the leash and walk Charlie.

No doubt about it, Charlie was Dad's dog. I mean, Charlie certainly tolerated Cal and me as we grew up. He was obedient whenever we took him on his afternoon walks. But inside, he'd move into another room away from us. Sure, he'd wag his tail at Mom as she'd put down his bowl of water. And Friday evenings, when she'd served a chicken for the Sabbath, Charlie would be far more expressive as she gave him the extra schmaltz. But it never lasted. When Dad was at work, Charlie would wait patiently on a scatter rug and ignore all of us. He never barked at the mailman, and left most of the other humans alone as they entered the door. But when he'd hear Dad close the garage, Charlie would jump up, move to the front door and bark wildly. When younger, Charlie would get up on his back legs, put his front paws on Dad's shoulders and lick Dad's face. In return, Dad would always be greeting Charlie first, then he'd nod to the rest of us. As Charlie would get down, Dad would kiss and then scratch Charlie's big blond head.

When Charlie died, sometime after I followed Cal to college, Dad fell into a deep funk. But after some months, he got another—this time a mutt—a Lab terrier mongrel. He called it Chuckles—in honor of Charlie, I guess. Chuckles was also good-natured, and, unlike Charlie, he was rotund, a bit swaybacked, and lower energy. Dad still took those morning walks. I suppose the two of them looked more fitting together—Dad no longer being shown up by a lean blond athletic type.

Without Cal and me at home, while Dad still worked, Mom walked Chuckles in the early afternoon. But Dad would take him out in the evenings and nights. All the dogs were always really Dad's. He loved his pets.

And once he retired, Dad was the one who walked Chuckles, almost always. He had his routes. Most mornings he'd go around a few blocks, so Chuckles could say good morning to everyone. He thought that, like Charlie, Chuckles needed a strong social life. This was in sharp contrast to himself. Dad never seemed to need more companionship than he got out of his dogs. He'd sit at the table with us, eating our meals. But aside from taking scraps and giving them to Charlie, I can't recall him having any sustained social communication with a living member of the household at the table.

Well, maybe that's a slight exaggeration, 'cause if we weren't respecting Mom, we'd know Dad wasn't going to tolerate it. But not much more. I know that sounds pretty extreme. Maybe I've forgotten a time or two. I'd have to check with Cal.

Even apart from mealtimes, I can't remember him talking to Mom *about* anything. I mean, you could hear a "yes" or a "no." Or some short answer to a question. And of course, there'd be the standard questions:

"Did you see Chuckles' leash?" or "Have you seen the car keys?" or "What'cha cooking, Rachel?"

Not that they weren't happy. He'd smile; they'd hug. Sometimes if the radio played just the right music they'd get up, laugh, and dance. But talk? Really talk? I doubt it. I think they never had a conversation. Not in front of us boys anyhow. Can you imagine my surprise hearing him talk to her after she passed? I'd come home for a holiday or something, and I'd hear him say things like, "Rachel, don't you concern yourself none anymore. All your boys, David, Cal, and me, we're truckin' just fine. They got themselves good jobs now. Just like you always wanted."

Another time it was about the garden: "Don't you be too worried about me anymore. I got the bulbs in just like you like, and the garden is going to be real pretty this year. You'll love it—we'll be able to look out the window and see all the flowers. Just you and me."

Well, I was so surprised that I called Cal first chance I had, and he could hardly believe it. He made me tell him the story two times before he accepted it as "real" information.

Big dogs may be fun, but they don't live long, most times. And sure enough, not long after Mom died, so did Chuckles. Chuckles's death just highlighted how alone Dad was. It marked the beginning of Dad's downturn.

He was inconsolable. 'Course, unlike when Mom died and Cal and I came home, neither of us thought about going home for Chuckles. Probably should have. Maybe Cal was too far away—I'm not exactly sure where he was that day we each got the call from Dad. As a journalist, he could have been sent anywhere. Maybe Cal was already in Libya, maybe he was just getting set to go. But I was in Chicago working for Sears. It took me a few weeks to realize how depressed Dad was. I mean, I'd call home in the morning and he wouldn't pick up. Even at noon he'd just say he had been sleeping— was just now getting up. It seemed like he'd never go out except to get food.

I got worried and asked for a transfer from Ohio to be nearer to Dad. I got it too. They set me up to manage the store in New Rochelle. Not the best place. Sort of an old store with problems, but just what I needed. I took an apartment in Larchmont. That gave me plenty of time to see him. At first, I'd get to his place and fix him breakfast so it'd be ready about an hour after sunup. Like Mom would have done. To fit his natural schedule. Like when he had a dog. But without a dog, he'd no interest in getting up. Even with me there. Since I had to go to work, I didn't even see him those mornings.

I changed my routine. Stopped going by in the morning and went by to make supper. At first Dad would just sit there. His once black hair now snow white. Usually unshaven. Always quiet. Happy to see me though—I could tell. He'd get up, sometimes even give me a hug and a pat on the back.

Then one day, out of the blue, he said it, "Son, I gotta get me a pet. My life isn't complete without me helping someone."

"Sure, let's get you a dog, Dad."

"I don't want a dog."

"What d'ya mean, you always had a dog."

"Too much responsibility."

"Well, we can go to the rescue and get one that's older. House-broken already. A dog will get you out of your funk."

"I don't think so."

I didn't listen. I went out and got him a mutt from the pound. It seemed to be a sure bet. But some days later, when I came one evening to make dinner, I noticed the dog wasn't in the room.

"So, where's the dog?"

"I told you, I didn't want a dog."

"Maybe I should have let you pick your own dog, Dad. You do need a pet. So let's go on Saturday. This time, you do the selecting. You said it yourself, 'I've always had a dog.' It'll get you out of the house, get you talking with the neighbors again."

"I never talked to neighbors. And I ain't starting now. I don't even know if I'd like them."

"You've walked your dogs for more than twenty years in this place. What do you mean you don't know the neighbors? That's impossible."

"I'll get my own damn pet."

And so, it was that one day the next week, I came over to cook dinner: pork and beans and salad. When I got there, I noticed that the kitchen was a bit cleaner than when I usually started my cooking. There were only a couple of dishes in the sink and no grease or crumbs on the counters. When I mentioned the cleanliness, my father just smiled. Then he added, "I got me some new responsibilities now, and I take 'em seriously."

That got me thinking about his needing a dog again. And after we were sitting down to eat, I raised it again.

"I thought you were going to pick out your own dog. When are we going to do that?" Dad just nodded in the direction of the bookshelf off to the left behind me. I knew he had a few books, including a couple on dogs. So I figured he was telling me he was reading up on breeds.

"Jesus, Dad. You don't need to *read* about them, just get one." Again, Dad didn't say anything. He just shrugged me off and again nodded toward the bookshelf. I was annoyed but didn't turn around.

After some more long silences, I picked up the dishes. Turning and getting up to put them in the sink, I couldn't miss the addition to the bookshelf.

"You got yourself a pet goldfish, Dad? Is this some sort of joke?"

"She's Charlemagne. And she ain't a goldfish. She's a sailfin molly."

"Sorrrrie!" I exhaled and took in his seriousness. "Well, so much for the housebreaking and dog walking."

A few days later, I arrived and Dad's welding gear was on the kitchen table. The rest of the kitchen was still clean. Dad still looked scruffy but seemed less depressed—almost alert. "Hey Dad, are you selling this gear?"

"Hell no, David. I'm using it."

I didn't think to ask for what. But over the next days the projects proliferated. First there was a ramp up the stairs to the front porch. I wondered about that. Dad certainly didn't seem headed for a wheelchair anytime soon. When I asked why he built it, he just shrugged. Soon thereafter, I found the welding gear outside, along with my old American Flyer red wagon.

My attempts at communication about the changing debris on the porch yielded no response. Of course, this aroused my curiosity. Over the next week, a rather extensive steel and glass project was being built as an attachment to my wagon. When it was done, it had a sealable top. It occupied the entire base of the wagon. A few days later, nary a trace of Charlemagne was left on the bookshelf.

"Where'd the molly go, Dad?"

"Front porch. Watching what's happening."

"Fish don't watch what's happening."

"Charlemagne does."

I got worried. My dad was always a bit different. But this was extreme. I was thinking of contacting Cal. He knew I was seeing Dad regularly, but he was so far away, he couldn't really get involved. So I let it go. And then, for about a week, maybe more, I couldn't get back to the house. I was dealing with complaints about customer service in the appliance department. That was the meat and potatoes for Sears, and Chicago had called about it. All I could do is phone. I'd ask how things were, and I'd get a one word answer. I hoped the calls were telling him I was there if he needed me.

A couple more weeks went by, and I got a call from Mrs. Polakoff's son-in-law. He and his wife had moved in after Mrs. Polakoff had died. Ed was worried that my father had lost his way. Neighbors noticed that Dad had returned to walking every morning, afternoon, and evening. They were concerned because he was wheeling his fish in an aquarium attached to an old wagon and apparently talking to the fish as if it were a dog while he walked the fish around the neighborhood. I told Ed I'd get back to him.

As I ratcheted up my worries about Dad, the customer-service problems had to be put on hold. I couldn't deal with two emergencies at once. First, I called Cal. But the call didn't go well. After the filial pleasantries and preliminaries, I remember something like this:

"Tell me again, why are you concerned, David?"

"Dad's walking his fish around the neighborhood and talking to it like a dog."

"Is he hurting or disturbing anyone? Destroying property?"

"No."

"Is he disoriented in other ways?"

"No."

"How does he possibly walk a live fish?"

"He built an aquarium. Welded it, you know, and then welded the whole contraption to my old wagon."

Perhaps Cal's silence reflected his absorption of this detail, but I rather think he was suppressing a laugh. "Well he surely doesn't exhibit dementia, does he?"

"No, probably not."

"Dad's walking his fish around the neighborhood hardly cuts it as a reason for me to get off assignment at this moment. Good luck David! And thanks for being there for us." Then he hung up.

I got to the house that night. Dad was well shaved, fully dressed, and in good spirits.

Digging into the tomato soup I'd made, I began, "Dad, I hear you are taking Charlemagne out for walks."

"Yup. She loves it."

"How do you know?"

"She's much more lively and less depressed. And her color is better." I put down my spoon and walked out the front door and checked. There was the fish, still atop her red American Flyer throne. The molly did seem perky, but I couldn't see a change in her color. I came back in.

"Dad, do you really think the fish is better off with the walks?"

"Of course. Fish are social animals. They live in schools. You know that. She's got to know her neighbors."

"But fish don't even live out here in air. They only know the world in water."

"Of course. Charles is in water. Always."

I hadn't heard him call her Charles before. It took me aback. Charles was legged, not finned.

"You mean Charlemagne?"

"'Course. Look, she needs her social time. You can't just isolate a pet."

"But her social time would be with other fish, under water."

Dad just sat there, taking this in. Then he said "Isn't there gonna be more than soup?"

"Aren't you concerned about what the neighbors think? I mean taking a fish for a walk could be seen as a sign of lunacy."

"I don't even know the neighbors. Fuck 'em. Why would I care if they thought I was crazy? What's for the rest of this meal? Stop giving me the fourth degree."

"We got tuna salad, and it's third degree." Then I dropped it. The next day I called Ed, told him not to worry, my Dad was doing fine, better than any time since my Mom died in fact. And I went back to my store's problems.

The weeks that followed were easy. Things went smoothly at Sears. Charlemagne was getting her socials. Dad was getting out and getting exercise. So what if he had some idiosyncrasies? He wasn't out to win the esteem of his neighbors.

But then one day, while working on a sales projection report, I got a call from the Mamaroneck police. "We've got your Dad. You've got to come down and get him."

"What? Is he locked up?"

"We didn't lock him up, we pulled him out of the Long Island Sound."

"Jesus, is he OK?"

"Well, he's a bit damp behind the ears. He may need a little care."

"But where? Was he swimming?"

"Just get down here, and then we'll discuss it. Be sure to bring him some dry clothes . . . Oh, and a warm blanket if you can."

So I picked up some dry stuff and went down to the police station. Dad was a sorry sight.

"What happened, Dad?"

"They left Charlemagne in the middle of the Sound. She's going to die if we don't pull her out."

The officer rolled her eyes. "Who the fuck is Charlemagne?"

"A fish," I replied.

"Well, your father was drifting off the Larchmont Manor Park shore. He was holding onto something that weighed him down. A crowd of people had gathered and were telling him to come back. He said he couldn't get out because of a wagon. Mr. Plixit jumped in to help him to shore, but he started fighting Mr. Plixit. Almost drowned him. They called the police, and we got him out. I don't know what this wagon crap is all about. You'd better make sure he gets into some kind of home—gets evaluated, if you know what I mean."

After Dad got on the dry clothes, we left the station and I got Dad's side of the story. Plixit wouldn't help him pull out the wagon and tried to force him to let it go.

"David, we've got to rescue Charlemagne. She's out beyond the gazebo. About ten feet, I think. We should be able to find her." He looked desperate. All the improvement I had witnessed was lost.

"Why'd you do it Dad? Why'd you put the wagon in the water?"

"You told me I had to. You were right. Charlemagne wasn't interested in her neighbor's dogs. She needed the sea."

So, of course we went to Abe's sporting goods, picked up a scuba mask, and then went to the Manor Park. As I stripped to my skivvies, I specified my conditions.

"Look Dad, I'm doing this for you. Not for Charlemagne. But you have to agree, if I save her, you don't go into the water with her anymore. Deal?"

"You help me get her, and it's a deal."

I looked into his eyes: he was sincere.

I waded in. It was cold, but bearable. There was a lot of seaweed and not much light. It took a good fifteen minutes or so to locate the wagon. It was only visible when the sun peeked out from the clouds for a minute and shone on the stainless-steel frame of the aquarium.

I dove down, found the handle, and struggled to get it to come toward the shore. Once it got close, I realized it was far too heavy to pull over the rocks. Luckily, a crowd had gathered around Dad, and when I got the wagon up on the first rocks, about half out of the water, they stared in amazement. I must have been a sight. Balding, graying at the temples, already with a beer belly more appropriate for someone twenty years older, pulling on a wagon handle over the barnacles. Dressed in my skivvies and a big black diving mask with a yellow breathing snorkel.

I looked at them and asked for some help. After a half a minute of hesitation, a couple of young guys pulled off their shoes and pants and came down into the water. The three of us were able to land that weird contraption welded onto my American Flyer. Once up on the grass, I inspected Charlemagne. She was quite alive.

The next day I began to look into nursing homes. I visited a few. What can I say? We all know what those places are like. I couldn't do it. But I'm a manager, someone who is supposed to think creatively. So I tried.

I put the ad on Craigslist.

Free room and board for dog walker who is willing to take elderly man on walks, call Sears in New Rochelle and ask for the store manager or dial extension 073.

The ad got a lot of bites. I interviewed about five or six of them and chose Debbie. She was sixty-seven, strong, healthy, and fourteen years younger than my father.

She cooked lasagna, meatloaf, sauces, desserts. A far better cook than I am. Dad put on weight again. They got along. I even heard them talking a few times. She walked with my father. Pretty soon she was walking most of the dogs in the neighborhood, and Dad went along. Charlemagne was still healthy, and I moved on.

When Sears offered to put me in charge of a K-Mart back in Ohio, I took it. It may not be my preferred reassignment, but it removed me from the everyday watch of my Dad. I worried less.

I was going to see Debbie and Dad about once a month. It would just be for an overnight, so I didn't witness all the day-to-day routines. Because I hadn't witnessed it or heard about it, I assumed Dad had given up some of the more bizarre behavior that had brought on the crisis.

But last time we got together, it was for a big shindig called by Dad for Charlemagne's third birthday. Cal even got there; flew in from somewhere abroad. There was cake and ice cream and Cal's imported prosecco. He also brought an unusual fancy and expensive fish food for Charlemagne. Charlemagne seemed pleased with her treat. Dad even swore he could see her wag her tail. Anyhow, after Cal presented Charlemagne with her birthday present, he popped open the prosecco, poured each of us a glass, and toasted the fish:

"Here's wishing you, and your master, a wonderful year of companionship!" We all assented and drank up.

Sotto voce, Debbie informed Cal and myself that we should get a second fish now, before Charlemagne's demise, "After all, what do you think the life expectancy of a goldfish is?"

"A molly," I corrected.

"Whatever." But she had a point. So I made the next toast.

"Happy birthday, Charlemagne. Here's hoping we find you a wonderful partner and tank mate to keep you social and happy during your fourth year." Dad did not take my toast well. He was dead set against my implication of another fish.

"What are you talking about, David? How can you expect some-one my age to take care of two pets?"

"Well, you'd have my help," Debbie pointed out.

"What do you mean you couldn't feed two fish?" chimed in Cal.

"It's not the feeding, Cal. It's the walking. I might not be able to build another tank or even if I could, I couldn't handle two tanks on that little wagon. What if Debbie gets sick or we're snow-bound? I can't do it."

Cal and I glanced at each other in surprise. This was the first we heard that Dad was still walking the fish. Anyone looking at us would have seen we were both horrified.

But before anything more could be added, Debbie said a second fish would take some pressure off; after all, it would let Charlemagne be social all the time, even on days she wasn't walked.

"I've heard with more than one fish in a tank, the more aggressive ones kill the others. What makes you think Charlemagne won't be eaten alive by your 'partner'?" countered Dad.

"Or even that Charlemagne might be the most aggressive?" I put in.

"Don't be ridiculous, David. Charlemagne is obviously not aggressive."

Taking out his phone, Cal said this was precisely what one could discover on the web. "Let's see now. Is the plural of 'mollys' *y-s* or *i-e-s*?"

"You're in the word business."

"Come on, bro, don't be a smartass—you know it's all video now. Ahh, *i-e-s*. Mollyfish.com, nifty. And there it is: I can click directly on 'tank mates,' what could be easier? Holy sheez! Debbie's right. Right here it says, your molly could be getting lonely! I can't believe it."

"Come on, Cal, let me see that," insisted Dad. Cal handed him the cell phone. Of course, Dad didn't have the right glasses on, but Debbie grabbed the phone and read it out loud. Then she got to the part about how some fish, including mollies, give birth to live, swim-ming babies. I was amazed.

"Yeah, but what about the aggression factor?" Dad asked.

"It discusses that too," continued Debbie. "Here it says mollies are very laid-back and easy to get along with. They're communal."

"Just like us," Dad said.

Cal and I glanced at each other, raised our eyebrows. I gave him a thumbs-up.

DIEM PERDIDI
Julie Otsuka

She remembers her name. She remembers the name of the president. She remembers the name of the president's dog. She remembers what city she lives in. And on which street. And in which house. *The one with the big olive tree where the road takes a turn.* She remembers what year it is. She remembers the season. She remembers the day on which you were born. She remembers the daughter who was born before you—*She had your father's nose, that was the first thing I noticed about her*—but she does not remember that daughter's name. She remembers the name of the man she did not marry—Frank—and she keeps his letters in a drawer by her bed. She remembers that you once had a husband, but she refuses to remember your ex-husband's name. *That man,* she calls him.

She does not remember how she got the bruises on her arms or going for a walk with you earlier this morning. She does not remember bending over, during that walk, and plucking a flower from a neighbor's front yard and slipping it into her hair. *Maybe your father will kiss me now.* She does not remember what she ate for dinner last night, or when she last took her medicine. She does not remember to drink enough water. She does not remember to comb her hair.

She remembers the rows of dried persimmons that once hung from the eaves of her mother's house in Berkeley. *They were the most beautiful shade of orange.* She remembers that your father loves peaches. She remembers that every Sunday morning, at ten, he takes her for a drive down to the sea in the brown car. She remembers that every evening, right before the eight o'clock news, he sets out two fortune cookies on a paper plate and announces to her that they are having a party. She remembers that on Mondays he comes home from the college at four, and if he is even five minutes late, she goes out to the gate and begins to wait for him. She remembers which bedroom is hers and which is his. She remembers that the bedroom that is now hers was once yours. She remembers that it wasn't always like this.

She remembers the first line of the song, "How High the Moon." She remembers the Pledge of Allegiance. She remembers her Social Security number. She remembers her best friend Jean's telephone number, even though Jean has been dead for six years. She remembers that Margaret is dead. She remembers that Betty is dead. She remembers that Grace has stopped calling. She remembers that her own mother died nine years ago, while spading the soil in her garden, and she misses her more and more every day. *It doesn't go away.* She remembers the number assigned to her family by the government right after the start of the war. *13611.* She remembers being sent away to the desert with her mother and brother during the fifth month of that war and taking her first ride on a train. She remembers the day they came home. *September 9, 1945.* She remembers the sound of the wind hissing through the sagebrush. She remembers the scorpions and red ants. She remembers the taste of dust.

Whenever you stop by to see her, she remembers to give you a big hug, and you are always surprised at her strength. She remembers to give you a kiss every time you leave. She remembers to tell you, at the end of every phone call, that the FBI will check up on you again soon. She remembers to ask you if you would like her to iron your blouse for you before you go out on a date. She remembers to smooth down your skirt. *Don't give it all away.* She remembers to brush aside a wayward strand of your hair. She does not remember eating lunch with you twenty minutes ago and suggests that you go out to Marie Callender's for sandwiches and pie. She does not remember that she herself once used to make the most beautiful pies with perfectly fluted crusts. She does not remember how to iron your blouse for you or when she began to forget. *Something's changed.* She does not remember what she is supposed to do next.

She remembers that the daughter who was born before you lived for half an hour and then died. *She looked perfect from the outside.* She remembers her mother telling her, more than once, *Don't you ever let anyone see you cry.* She remembers giving you your first bath on your third day in the world. She remembers that you were a very fat baby. She remembers that your first word was *No.* She remembers picking apples in a field with Frank many years ago in the rain. *It was the best day of my life.* She remembers that the first time she met him she was so nervous she forgot her own address. She remembers wearing too much lipstick. She remembers not sleeping for days.

When you drive past Hesse Park, she remembers being asked to leave her exercise class by her teacher after being in that class for more than ten years. *I shouldn't have talked so much.* She remembers touching her toes and doing windmills and jumping jacks on the freshly mown grass. She remembers being the highest kicker in her class. She does not remember how to use the "new" coffee maker, which is now three years old, because it was bought after she began to forget. She does not remember asking your father, ten minutes ago, if today is Sunday, or if it is time to go for her ride. She does not remember where she last put her sweater or how long she has been sitting in her chair. She does not always remember how to get out of that chair, and so you gently push down on the footrest and offer her your hand, which she does not always remember to take. *Go away,* she sometimes says. Other times, she just says, *I'm stuck.* She does not remember saying to you, the other night, right after your father left the room, *He loves me more than I love him.* She does not remember saying to you, a moment later, *I can hardly wait until he comes back.*

She remembers that when your father was courting her, he was always on time. She remembers thinking that he had a nice smile. *He still does.* She remembers that when they first met he was engaged to another woman. She remembers that that other woman was white. She remembers that that other woman's parents did not want their daughter to marry a man who looked like the gardener. She remembers that the winters were colder back then, and that there were days on which you actually had to put on a coat and scarf. She remembers her mother bowing her head every morning at the altar and offering her ancestors a bowl of hot rice. She remembers the smell of incense and pickled cabbage in the kitchen. She remembers that her father always wore nice shoes. She remembers that the night the FBI came for him, he and her mother had just had another big fight. She remembers not seeing him again until after the end of the war.

She does not always remember to trim her toenails, and when you soak her feet in the bucket of warm water, she closes her eyes and leans back in her chair and reaches out for your hand. *Don't give up on me.* She does not remember how to tie her shoelaces, or fasten the hooks on her bra. She does not remember that she has been wearing her favorite blue blouse for five days in a row. She does not remember your age. *Just wait till you have children of your own,* she says to you, even though you are now too old to do so.

She remembers that after the first girl was born and then died, she sat in the yard for days, just staring at the roses by the pond. *I didn't know what else to do.* She remembers that when you were born, you, too, had your father's long nose. *It was as if I'd given birth to the same girl twice.* She remembers that you are a Taurus. She remembers that your birthstone is green. She remembers to read you your horoscope from the newspaper whenever you come over to see her. *Someone you were once very close to may soon reappear in your life,* she tells you. She does not remember reading you that same horoscope five minutes ago or going to the doctor with you last week after you discovered a bump on the back of her head. *I think I fell.* She does not remember telling the doctor that you are no longer married, or giving him your number and asking him to please call. She does not remember leaning over and whispering to you, the moment he stepped out of the room, *I think he'll do.*

She remembers another doctor asking her, fifty years ago, minutes after the first girl was born and then died, if she wanted to donate the baby's body to science. *He said she had a very unusual heart.* She remembers being in labor for thirty-two hours. She remembers being too tired to think. *So I told him yes.* She remembers driving home from the hospital in the sky-blue Chevy with your father and neither one of them saying a word. She remembers knowing she'd made a big mistake. She does not remember what happened to the baby's body and worries that it might be stuck in a jar. She does not remember why they didn't just bury her. *I wish she were under a tree.* She remembers wanting to bring her flowers every day.

She remembers that even as a young girl you said you did not want to have children. She remembers that you hated wearing dresses. She remembers that you never played with dolls. She remembers that the first time you bled you were thirteen years old and wearing bright yellow pants. She remembers that your childhood dog was named Shiro. She remembers that you once had a cat named Gasoline. She remembers that you had two turtles named Turtle. She remembers that the first time she and your father took you to Japan to meet his family you were eighteen months old and just beginning to speak. She remembers leaving you with his mother in the tiny silkworm village in the mountains while she and your father traveled across the island for ten days. *I worried about you the whole time.* She remembers that when they came back, you did not know who she was and that for many days afterwards you would not speak to her, you would only whisper in her ear.

She remembers that the year you turned five you refused to leave the house without tapping the door frame three times. She remembers that you had a habit of clicking your teeth repeatedly, which drove her up the wall. She remembers that you could not stand it when different-colored foods were touching on the plate. *Everything had to be just so.* She remembers trying to teach you to read before you were ready. She remembers taking you to Newberry's to pick out patterns and fabric and teaching you how to sew. She remembers that every night, after dinner, you would sit down next to her at the kitchen table and hand her the bobby pins one by one as she set the curlers in her hair. She remembers that this was her favorite part of the day. *I wanted to be with you all the time.*

She remembers that you were conceived on the first try. She remembers that your brother was conceived on the first try. She remembers that your other brother was conceived on the second try. *We must not have been paying attention.* She remembers that a palm reader once told her that she would never be able to bear children because her uterus was tipped the wrong way. She remembers that a blind fortune-teller once told her that she had been a man in her past life, and that Frank had been her sister. She remembers that everything she remembers is not necessarily true. She remembers the horse-drawn garbage carts on Ashby, her first pair of crepe-soled shoes, scattered flowers by the side of the road. She remembers that the sound of Frank's voice always made her feel calmer. She remembers that every time they parted he turned around and watched her walk away. She remembers that the first time he asked her to marry him she told him she wasn't ready. She remembers that the second time she said she wanted to wait until she was finished with school. She remembers walking along the water with him one warm summer evening on the boardwalk and being so happy she could not remember her own name. She remembers not knowing that it wouldn't be like this with any of the others. She remembers thinking she had all the time in the world.

She does not remember the names of the flowers in the yard whose names she has known for years. *Roses? Daffodils? Immortelles?* She does not remember that today is Sunday, and she has already gone for her ride. She does not remember to call you, even though she always says that she will. She remembers how to play *Clair de Lune* on the piano. She remembers how to play *Chopsticks* and scales. She remembers not to talk to telemarketers when they call on the telephone. *We're not interested.* She remembers her grammar. *Just between you and me.* She remembers her manners. She remembers to say thank you and please. She remembers to wipe herself every time she uses the toilet. She remembers to flush. She remembers to turn her wedding ring around whenever she pulls on her silk stockings. She remembers to reapply her lipstick every time she leaves the house. She remembers to put on her anti-wrinkle cream every night before climbing into bed. *It works while you sleep.* In the morning, when she wakes, she remembers her dreams. *I was walking through a forest. I was swimming in a river. I was looking for Frank in a city I did not know and no one would tell me where he was.*

On Halloween day, she remembers to ask you if you are going out trick-or-treating. She remembers that your father hates pumpkin. *It's all he ate in Japan during the war.* She remembers listening to him pray, every night, when they first got married, that he would be the one to die first. She remembers playing marbles on a dirt floor in the desert with her brother and listening to the couple at night on the other side of the wall. *They were at it all the time.* She remembers the box of chocolates you brought back to her after your honeymoon in Paris. "But will it last?" you asked her. She remembers her own mother telling her, "The moment you fall in love with someone, you are lost."

She remembers that when her father came back after the war, he and her mother fought even more than they had before. She remembers that he would spend entire days shopping for shoes in San Francisco while her mother scrubbed other people's floors. She remembers that some nights he would walk around the block three times before coming into the house. She remembers that one night he did not come in at all. She remembers that when your own husband left you, five years ago, you broke out in hives all over your body for weeks. She remembers thinking he was trouble the moment she met him. *A mother knows.* She remembers keeping that thought to herself. *I had to let you make your own mistakes.*

She remembers that, of her three children, you were the most delightful to be with. She remembers that your younger brother was so quiet she sometimes forgot he was there. *He was like a dream.* She remembers that her own brother refused to carry anything with him onto the train except for his rubber toy truck. *He wouldn't let me touch it.* She remembers her mother killing all the chickens in the yard the day before they left. She remembers her fifth-grade teacher, Mr. Martello, asking her to stand up in front of the class so everyone could tell her goodbye. She remembers being given a silver heart pendant by her next-door neighbor, Elaine Crowley, who promised to write but never did. She remembers losing that pendant on the train and being so angry she wanted to cry. *It was my first piece of jewelry.*

She remembers that one month after Frank joined the Air Force he suddenly stopped writing her letters. She remembers worrying that he'd been shot down over Korea or taken hostage by guerrillas in the jungle. She remembers thinking about him every minute of the day. *I thought I was losing my mind.* She remembers learning from a friend one night that he had fallen in love with somebody else. She remembers asking your father the next day to marry her. *"Shall we go get the ring?" I said to him.* She remembers telling him, *It's time.*

When you take her to the supermarket, she remembers that coffee is Aisle Two. She remembers that Aisle Three is milk. She remembers the name of the cashier in the express lane who always gives her a big hug. *Diane.* She remembers the name of the girl at the flower stand who always gives her a single broken-stemmed rose. She remembers that the man behind the meat counter is Big Lou. "Well, hello, gorgeous," he says to her. She does not remember where her purse is, and begins to panic until you remind her that she has left it at home. *I don't feel like myself without it.* She does not remember asking the man in line behind her whether or not he was married. She does not remember him telling her, rudely, that he was not. She does not remember staring at the old woman in the wheelchair by the melons and whispering to you, *I hope I never end up like that.* She remembers that the huge mimosa tree that once stood next to the cart corral in the parking lot is no longer there. *Nothing stays the same.* She remembers that she was once a very good driver. She remembers failing her last driver's test three times in a row. *I couldn't remember any of the rules.* She remembers that the day after her father left them, her mother sprinkled little piles of salt in the corner of every room to purify the house. She remembers that they never spoke of him again.

She does not remember asking your father, when he comes home from the pharmacy, what took him so long, or who he talked to, or whether or not the pharmacist was pretty. She does not always remember his name. She remembers graduating from high school with high honors in Latin. She remembers how to say, "I came, I saw, I conquered." *Veni, vidi, vici.* She remembers how to say, "I have lost the day." *Diem perdidi.* She remembers the words for "I'm sorry" in

Japanese, which you have not heard her utter in years. She remembers the words for "rice" and "toilet." She remembers the words for "Wait." *Chotto matte kudasai.* She remembers that a white-snake dream will bring you good luck. She remembers that it is bad luck to pick up a dropped comb. She remembers that you should never run to a funeral. She remembers that you shout the truth down into a well.

She remembers going to work, like her mother, for the rich white ladies up in the hills. She remembers Mrs. Tindall, who insisted on eating lunch with her every day in the kitchen instead of just leaving her alone. She remembers Mrs. Edward deVries, who fired her after one day. *"Who taught you how to iron?" she asked me.* She remembers that Mrs. Cavanaugh would not let her go home on Saturdays until she had baked an apple pie. She remembers Mrs. Cavanaugh's husband, Arthur, who liked to put his hand on her knee. She remembers that he sometimes gave her money. She remembers that she never refused. She remembers once stealing a silver candlestick from a cupboard but she cannot remember whose it was. She remembers that they never missed it. She remembers using the same napkin for three days in a row. She remembers that today is Sunday, which six days out of seven is not true.

When you bring home the man you hope will become your next husband, she remembers to take his jacket. She remembers to offer him coffee. She remembers to offer him cake. She remembers to thank him for the roses. *So you like her?* she asks him. She remembers to ask him his name. *She's my firstborn, you know.* She remembers, five minutes later, that she has already forgotten his name, and asks him again what it is. *That's my brother's name,* she tells him. She does not remember talking to her brother on the phone earlier that morning—*He promised me he'd call*—or going for a walk with you in the park. She does not remember how to make coffee. She does not remember how to serve cake.

She remembers sitting next to her brother many years ago on a train to the desert and fighting about who got to lie down on the seat. She remembers hot white sand, the wind on the water, someone's voice telling her, *Hush, it's all right.* She remembers where she was the day the men landed on the moon. She remembers the day they learned that Japan had lost the war. *It was the only time I ever saw my mother cry.* She remembers the day she learned that Frank had married somebody else. *I read about it in the paper.* She remembers the letter she got from him not long after, asking if he could please see her. *He said he'd made a mistake.* She remembers writing him back, "It's too late." She remembers marrying your father on an unusually warm day in December. She remembers having their first fight, three months later, in March. *I threw a chair.* She remembers that he comes home from the college every Monday at four. She remembers that she is forgetting. She remembers less and less every day.

When you ask her your name, she does not remember what it is. *Ask your father. He'll know.* She does not remember the name of the president. She does not remember the name of the president's dog. She does not remember the season. She does not remember the day or the year. She remembers the little house on San Luis Avenue that she first lived in with your father. She remembers her mother leaning over the bed she once shared with her brother and kissing the two of them goodnight. She remembers that as soon as the first girl was born she knew that something was wrong. *She didn't cry.* She remembers holding the baby in her arms and watching her go to sleep for the first and last time in her life. She remembers that they never buried her. She remembers that they did not give her a name. She remembers that the baby had perfect fingernails and a very unusual heart. She remembers that she had your father's long nose. She remembers knowing at once that she was his. She remembers beginning to bleed two days later when she came home from the hospital. She remembers your father catching her in the bathroom as she began to fall. She remembers a desert sky at sunset. *It was the most beautiful shade of orange.* She remembers scorpions and red ants. She remembers the taste of dust. She remembers once loving someone more than anyone else. She remembers giving birth to the same girl twice. She remembers that today is Sunday, and it is time to go for her ride, and so she picks up her purse and puts on her lipstick and goes out to wait for your father in the car.

DEMENTED

Lauren Francis-Sharma

"Your hands feel like chalk, child," she said. "It's no wonder you couldn't keep that boy's father. You think anybody wants you touching them with those hard hands?" My mother slid her arms beneath the pink blanket, gripping the cushion of the loveseat with its canvas slipcover before closing her eyes.

I sometimes convinced myself that what my mother said was not what she would have said before the diagnosis. I sometimes convinced myself that that woman with the pursed mouth spraying words like old vomit was not my mother. But some things felt too familiar for me to be fully convinced.

"Ma, my hands are hard because I have to wash them all the time." My mother wasn't listening. We'd found her old cassettes and a boom box with a tape deck. Al Green always quieted her. "I wash them before I make your food. Before I lift you from the bed. After I change your diaper. After I get poop on my fingers." I wanted her to hear me, but instead she rubbed her face, the mustache she'd once tweezed on Sunday nights thick and curly.

Ma had been a school principal, a church organist, a woman who thumped me with her red-leather Bible if I didn't wake for school. She wore cockatoo brooches at the neck of her blouses and double-girdled her behind because she didn't want to "tempt the masses." My mother was a sanctified, respectable woman, who had put herself through college by the time I was seven, who had earned her master's degree by the time I was fifteen. And when Ma was accepted into a doctoral program and Daddy did what was expected of a man like him, Ma spared him the shame of divorce and instead sent his mistress a hand-written note about what to do at nights when he choked in his sleep: *Just knock him on the forehead as hard as you can,* she wrote.

Demented. Dementia. "De-" used to convey something is lacking or without. "Mens," meaning sense or mind. *Demens.* Which to me sounded very much like "demons," for my mother seemed often a woman possessed. Possessed by an uncertainty that had never been hers before. My Ma, who was once so certain of herself that she rewired our house for stereo sound with only a Radio Shack manual; my Ma, who could make it from Baltimore to Brooklyn in three hours driving a Toyota Tercel. This mother of mine didn't remember her own name.

I had been an only child and was raising a boy alone when Ma came to live with us. I didn't want to take care of her. This was not something one said. And yet, I didn't want anyone to say that I had not.

Ma had always been honest about the burdens of motherhood. It was an accepted truth in our home that her only child was hard work. Too much work. I had big hair that needed to be tamed and a big mouth that needed to be heard. Ma was always dutiful. It was her job "to raise me right," and my job "to behave right." When I told her about my pregnancy and my intention to quit law school, she told me I'd been her greatest cross and would also be her greatest failure.

Who knew she would be mine too?

"Children eat brains, you know. What's that show you used to watch? Little aliens implanting themselves in people's stomachs and killing their hosts," she'd said. "You're gonna wake up and your mind won't be your own. You'll feel hungry when that baby's hungry. You won't remember what you want or what you used to enjoy, somebody will ask you what makes you happy and you won't know. You'll see."

"Raising my child will be an honor. I am not you," I told her.

"You believe that?"

"Which part?"

She laughed and told me to call the clinic.

My mother's laughter used to embarrass me. She didn't laugh

often, but when she did, it was hearty and throaty. My childhood friend, Simone, once said that my mother's laugh was "uncouth." When I asked Ma what that meant, she said it meant "ghetto."

"That debauched mother of hers must've told her that," Ma said. "I'mma bake them a cake and put a big Black laughing face on it." My mother giggled herself to sleep when she returned from leaving it on Simone's doorstep.

"Get it away!" Ma waved her hands about her face. "I ate already!" Often Ma did not remember to eat, did not remember having eaten. Every morning before I took Charles to school, Ma protested when I set her blue plastic breakfast plate down before her. "You're trying to make me fat like you!"

I pushed the plate toward her chest. "Yes, Ma, I gained weight." I had put on thirty-six pounds since she took over the first floor of my house. I couldn't afford new clothes, so zippers remained unzipped, buttons remained unbuttoned. "Nine pounds for each year you've been here." I'd eaten Charles's lunch snacks every night after Ma lost the battle against sleep, and then another handful of Utz crackers and a hunk of cheddar cheese, each time she'd wake during the night. "I am very happy to have something in my mouth to stop me from screaming."

Ma glared as if disappointed in *my* choice of words.

A year after she moved in, Ma began to shout each evening at sundown. They told me this would happen, and yet this was when I began to dislike my own mother's face. A monstrous sunken mask, it seemed to me, cheeks sagging like deflated balloons, jowls plunging like her memory, a quicksand in which lost things would never be found. And in the whites behind her black pupils, there seemed no life remaining, only the reflection of my own soured and exhausted expression.

My childhood friend Simone had a mother with a face from a Spiegel's catalogue. Her name was also Simone. This name recycling was something my mother said one did when one thought too much of oneself. Ma said Ms. Simone thought too much of herself. Ms. Simone was the sort of woman the boys on corner posts whispered about, the kind of woman who wore lipstick the same red as the Porsche 911 pictured on my bedroom posters. Ms. Simone had sharp Nordic features but her skin shone the color of Werther's butterscotch. "A fine woman," my father said once while Ma plated his food. My mother didn't disagree, but she made sure to give Daddy only one dumpling with his chicken that night.

Simone's father worked as an engineer in Trinidad. He assisted the United States government with building a winding road along his country's northwest coast. When he arrived in the States, he couldn't secure a better job than hauling parts at Union Carbide on the night shift. He spoke three languages, and Ms. Simone expected she would have a *Good Housekeeping* kind of life. After she realized her husband would come to nothing much, Ms. Simone took to having an affair with a bearded Frenchman who taught physics at Hopkins. This ended when Simone's father left a buffed machete on the passenger seat of the professor's restored BMW with a note that read: "Made in Trinidad and Tobago."

Outside of receiving Ma's initial diagnosis, I found myself most surprised when Ms. Simone began her weekly visits. She drove on Sundays from her retirement townhome in Pennsylvania to the suburbs of Washington, DC. Together, my mother and Ms. Simone watched Lifetime Television. Ms. Simone clapped for the women who ran their husbands off roads, talking to the television or to my mother, I couldn't quite tell. My little house smelled of Chanel No. 5 long after she left. I found those visits strange but also comforting and chalked them up to Ma's smiling cake having been delicious.

"You should call Little Simone," Ms. Simone said each week before she left. Ms. Simone was older than Ma by ten years, but time had been more agreeable with her. Her hands trembled a bit, the webbing around her eyes contracted when she grinned, and when she spoke her tongue took a bit more time hearing the words in her head, but there was no denying her now quiet beauty. "I'm sure she'd like to tell you some things."

I hadn't spoken to "Little Simone" in over twenty years. I didn't tell Ms. Simone that I followed her daughter's posts on Instagram.

That I thought that except for the unfortunate loss of her natural eyebrows, Little Simone was just as cute as when we were girls. I told myself that speaking to Simone would remind me of my mother's better days and make the pain of losing her worse, but I knew it was more than that.

"I can't come over no more," Little Simone told me one early summer's day in the alley behind my house. Someone had left their hose running, and I recalled the sound of trickling water, like a brook babbling. "My dad said you can't never come over again either."

We were thirteen, and we'd been spending every Saturday night at each other's homes since we were four years old. We had shared soggy fried chicken television dinners, took baths in my mother's rusted tub, French-kissed the same big-headed boys, hated the same stuck-up girls.

"It doesn't matter whether it's a boy or a girl or a dog. The heart makes no distinctions like that," my mother had said.

That summer my mother was the kindest she'd ever been to me. She told me I was better off without Simone, and Ma left me alone to cry in the peace of my bedroom with only the blue glowing light of Space Invaders to feed my crushed spirit. It was the hottest summer on record, and the fan in the window pulled and pushed warm air. When I emerged, two inches taller in the fall of my freshmen year, I was a girl hell-bent on proving Simone Sanders and her roti-eating father wrong about me. I studied my way out of the city's best public high school and then went on to the Ivy League. I was near the top of my class, when in my second year of law school, I met a boy who was more likely to have married a Simone than a me. A boy whose stepfather had a house on the Vineyard, a boy who never knew I had his son. Ma said she would not help take care of my baby. I told myself she deserved to live her life as she wished. But I was angry. As I pumped breastmilk into bottles and shuttled Charles between day-cares, Ma learned to swim, took karate, studied French.

"You only study French if you plan on going to France."

"Maybe I'll go to France," she'd said.

"You're never going to France."

I was sometimes an awful child to my mother.

As a grandmother, Ma offered only what was needed and nothing more. Charles was seven years old the first time I had to call Ma for assistance. I was home sick with the flu. Charles couldn't find his violin in the music room at school and missed his ride home. I had enrolled Charles in one of those fancy private schools like Simone once attended, with rolling hills and white people who traveled to Utah for skiing on long weekends. The gap between the tuition and the aid they offered was so wide I thought every month I'd drown in it, but I had pieced together a life for Charles and me that, at a far enough distance, looked much like the life I would have had if I had done it all the right way.

I regretted needing to call Ma. I knew she'd sashay herself onto that campus and shatter the suburban mom image I'd carefully culti-vated with her Baltimore City church-lady air. I told Ma to wait until aftercare was almost ended, to park in the lot and hike up the hill to sign out Charles. It would be easier, I had said. Ma told me her knee was swollen and that she'd be picking up Charles the way everyone else picked up their grandchildren. So I had to tell her how to man-age the carpool circle, how she mustn't be on her phone, or let her car idle, how she must make sure to use her emergency brake when she stopped on the steep hill.

"I'm not a goddamn child!" she screamed.

In all the years I'd taken my mother's words on the chin, she had never once cursed at me. As a principal, she told her kids if they had to resort to cursing, then they either didn't know the Lord or didn't know enough words. And she'd set them on the magic quilt in a quiet corner and make them choose between the Bible and the Oxford.

I should have known something was wrong, but I didn't think much of it until after she called me from the school.

"I hit somebody. And now he's calling the police."

"The police? Who did you hit?"

"Some man in a fucking Mercedes Benz who's cursing at me like I crucified Jesus!"

"Did you get his name? Did you hit him from the rear?"

"No. Head on. And the boy in his front seat didn't have a seatbelt on. That's not my goddamn fault."

They took away her license. She'd had more accidents than I'd known. One in New York City, another in Virginia Beach, two in Pennsylvania. Baltimore Gas & Electric had turned off her lights. Her taxes had gone unpaid. She'd been sending money to a sweet-talking Nigerian prince in Trenton. I'd hoped it was a benign tumor, that she could be fixed up, made right again, but after the diagnosis, three times checked, I knew there was nothing that could be made right ever again.

"You got no business looking at me like that!" I'd cracked open the bathroom window for fresh air while sponge-bathing her. A neighbor, walking her Cavachon, looked up, as if to ensure that Ma was being treated well. I wanted to scream out to that nosy woman that Ma wasn't the one who needed to be saved.

I turned to Ma. "Who's gonna look at you if I don't?" I said.

Daddy came to visit Ma once. She seemed to remember him and repeated the story, over and again, of Daddy not knowing the difference between a cucumber and a zucchini. Before he moved out, she'd embarrassed him at a cocktail party thrown by the Baltimore City school superintendent. It seemed the story embarrassed him still. Ma told him he was a man-baby, and when he stopped speaking and his big body sunk into my loveseat, Ma didn't care about his quiet, didn't notice when he left.

But Ma always noticed when Ms. Simone arrived. My mother smiled and reached for words that sounded feathery on her lips. I made sure on those days that her still-thick hair was curled, framing her face like a doily, and that I creamed her hands so they glistened when Ms. Simone reached for them.

One Sunday as Ms. Simone readied to leave, I thanked her again for not forgetting about Ma, for it seemed everyone else had.

"Your mother was everything I wanted," and then Ms. Simone's voice trailed off at "to be."

After Ms. Simone left, Charles fed Ma chopped chicken breast from his plate. I hadn't told him I had become too frightened to feed her, that my stomach soured when drool fell from the left side of her face, that I disliked watching the way she chewed. The chicken was over-cooked and I made a big fuss about it, moving about the kitchen so as to avoid the feeding. The nighttime aide hadn't yet arrived, so Charles kept Ma busy with a story about a boy at school who had tied a shirt around Charles's neck like a noose. Charles didn't tell Ma how he'd cried, how I'd held him in the back of my car, incensed that those white boys might've smelled that barely-keeping-it-together scent I'd passed on to him. Charles told Ma that I'd scolded the boy's mother, telling her that nooses weren't playthings for Black boys. "Grandma, she sounded just like you," he said.

My mother smiled, removed the chicken from her mouth, setting it on tablecloth. "That Simone's got big beautiful nipples. The color of baked peach cobbler," she said.

Charles stared at his grandmother, not certain he'd heard her correctly.

"This is the disease, Charles. This is not Grandma talking." I'd told him this, many times before. The disease, always it was the disease. Charles blushed then went to his room to finish his studies.

That night I found Little Simone on Facebook Messenger and asked if I could call her the next day.

I shared an office with another paralegal, a Russian woman who spoke in whispers to her imprisoned daughter each day at noon. Most days I left for lunch before her call, but when Simone answered the phone with a woman's voice I did not know, I found myself thinking only of how much I regretted that we hadn't seen each other grow into women. Simone told me all the things about her life that her mother had often mentioned. That she taught nursing, that her husband was an accountant, that her children both had black belts. I listened until I found enough quiet between us to ask why she stopped being my friend. I was crying ancient tears by then, feeling an old heartbreak like new. The Russian called me something that sounded like "sooka" and stared at me, with the phone to her head, her daughter on the other end crying too. I firmed my voice, as I explained to Little Simone, that the strain of taking care of Ma had left me overly emotional. That it was just a phase.

Simone said she understood, said she was sorry again.

Everyone was always sorry.

"My dad said that on the nights your mother played organ at the church she would drive down our street, park her car in front of our house, and stare into the window. You remember that my room was at the front, right?" Simone's bedroom carpet had been a cream-colored shag that never showed dirt. Each time I returned from her house, I'd try and convince Ma to take off her shoes in our bedrooms too. "My dad said your mother was a pervert."

Simone's father was crazy, and everyone knew it. He'd once choked Ms. Simone until she passed out, had set their basement on fire with some chemistry experiment gone wrong, had cursed out the mailman when he'd put someone else's mail in his box. I reminded Simone of all this.

"My mother was worried about you. Your mother wasn't attentive. You know that's all it was," I said.

"You remember what you used to call your mother? S-O-S?" she said. "Selfish ole Sally. She was *not* concerned about my welfare."

I had worked decades as a litigation paralegal. I knew how to think on my feet. Yet I heard myself quiet, for inside I was roiling, humiliated. What *had* my mother been doing at the front of their house? I tried to think of all the nights Simone had slept over, the time my mother helped Simone insert her first tampon so we could swim at the water park. Had my mother always been thinking of Little Simone in *that* way?

That night when my mother fought the nurse at bath time, she called out for me. I let the nurse put her to bed. The sound of the cotton socks encasing her cracked feet made me feel guilty. I should have lotioned her heels, painted her toenails in the purple she once favored. But I needed time to put the armor back on so that I could secure my mother's name in my own head. She had warned me many years earlier that I would need to protect my mind. I didn't think I'd have to protect it from her.

That night I realized I hadn't hugged my mother in something like four years. Hadn't kissed her in close to three. I wondered how long it'd been since she'd kissed me, hugged me. The answer seemed irrelevant. Everything about how I felt seemed irrelevant.

I called Simone again. "There's something you're not saying."

I had pulled Simone's first tooth, we'd won our neighborhood jacks tournament three summers in a row, had gotten lost on our Big Wheels in the woods and hugged each other the whole night hoping they'd come looking for us. But our parents didn't know we were missing.

"Sometimes at nights, your mother would come over." She said this as if she knew she'd have to one day say it.

"Ma came over to your house?"

"My mother told me if I ever told my dad that your Ma was there, she'd give into my father's demands to put me in public school."

"Wait. Your mother was home but not your father? What was my mother doing there?"

Charles moved about the kitchen, pretending he wasn't listening.

"Your mother would sit across from mine at the dining room table and when they thought I was asleep on the sofa, they'd go up into my parents' bedroom." Simone paused and I found myself unwilling to fill in the blank. "My mother sprayed Chanel No. 5 after your mother left."

"That's not true," I said.

I put Simone on hold and instructed Charles to check on Ma. She was knocking her fists on the tub again. The nurse had raised her voice. After I heard him walking up the stairs, I held the phone to my chest and wondered if my mother had allowed Ms. Simone to lie to her husband about why she had been watching their house?

"Before she got sick, your Ma would drive to Pennsylvania every Friday night and my mother would follow her in her car, down the I-70 on Sundays, and stay with her until Tuesday," Simone continued.

Ma had often told me that she was too tired to drive the forty-five minutes for Charles's Sunday soccer matches, that there was too much arthritis in her knees to sit on bleachers during his Saturday basketball games.

"Four nights, every week?"

I remembered little of Ma's early retirement years except thinking I didn't wish to be a lonely old Black woman like her. That I hated how her breasts sagged, how her skin soured more quickly when she perspired. Who would love her now, I remembered thinking? That's when I first searched for Charles's father on Facebook. He was married to a woman who could have been my sister. Same complexion, same wide face, same flat chest. His wife was a gynecologist. He was a consultant at Goldman Sachs. They lived on the Upper East Side in an apartment overlooking the park I'd once dreamt of rollerblading through. They had two girls. Both with bad teeth that I knew would be straightened in the same number of years it took their beautiful father to follow me back on Twitter, to ask why I'd dropped out of school. "My mother was sick," I'd lied.

"My mother and your mother, they love each other," Simone said.

Simone said "love" like this was a thing I understood. Like this was a thing Ma remembered and wanted, like this was a thing that held the power to make Ma new, to make my life new. I thought of all Ma's regrets, all mine, culminating into that one horrific moment on the phone with Simone where I denied knowing that Ma's life was never as she wanted, where I denied knowing that this was true for me too. I heard Simone smile, like she was happy for my mother, sad for hers, like she thought that me knowing of this love between them offered me relief as I cared for a woman who'd always done her duty. And I convinced myself that God would be more merciful to me.

CASTING STONES
Julia Tagliere

CHECK-IN

Ginger, all blond wig and movie-star sunglasses, thirty-year-old implants hanging on for dear life to a scrawny eighty-five-year-old chest, is not my new roommate's real name. She flirts with Matt the Certified Nursing Assistant (Our Cruise Director) during her daily sponge baths and bursts into Hollywood show tunes at odd hours. She claims to be a former Rockette, now wheelchair-bound, but her pink-chenille-slippered toes tap constantly, begging for dance partners. Sometimes I think putting vivacious Ginger in with me is my extra punishment for slipping up, for letting myself blink when I woke up and saw Matt raping my former roommate, Mrs. Margaret O'Brien (her real name) the last time. Maybe it was coincidence, but the next morning, Margaret was gone.

I'm sure you're thinking I should've said something the first time—is it really two years ago now? Well, I *did* say something. But if Charles, my own son, didn't believe me, why would anyone else? It took seven calls for him even to return my message.

"Listen, Mother," he'd said, sighing. "First it was having to share a room, then the cheap bedding, then the bad food, and now this? I mean, why would anybody—are you sure you're not just making up stories to get me to pull you out of there?"

I tried to slam the phone down but it slipped from my fingers. Charles's voice drifted up from the receiver on the floor; he didn't even realize I was no longer there.

"I've told you, Mother," he said, "I can't take care of you myself. This is the only place you can afford, so you're going to have to get used to it."

I tried clenching my hands into fists but gave up at pathetic little Cs. *Whose fault was it I couldn't afford better?*

The first time Matt "visited" Margaret, I'd pretended to be asleep. But, leaving her a still-none-the-wiser de facto turnip, he'd crept into bed with me after, smelling of beer and sweat. Too shocked even to scream, I shook so violently I wet my diaper. When it leaked, he rolled right off me; I made a mental note for future reference.

"Jesus Christ, you're disgusting," he said, slurring his words. He grabbed a corner of my blanket and began rubbing at his crotch. I fumbled for the call button, pressing it over and over, but no one came. I found out later he'd unplugged it.

Matt grunted and lay still beside me. Then he climbed out of my bed and pulled up his scrubs. He went to our bathroom; I heard water running. He returned with a washcloth and swiped at my blanket.

When Matt pulled the call button from my grasp, I opened my mouth to scream. He covered my face with one of his big hands; it smelled of antiseptic soap and lighter fluid. He whispered in my ear.

"You say anything, and you're next."

I called Charles again the next morning, and the next. On the seventh day, I stopped trying. That was the day I turned to stone.

DINNER AND A SHOW

Today must be Thursday, because Ted the Piano Man, he of the musical-note-dotted red bowtie, is here, bludgeoning the keys of the scarred old baby grand in our snot-yellow-hued lobby (the Sunflower Room).

When Charles still visited me every week, I almost looked forward to Thursdays. For that single hour each week, we could approximate a normal mother-son relationship. But before the end of the first year, not even a full one since his father's death, Charles had emptied our home, sold the contents ("I told you, Mother, the money can't be in your name, it'll screw up Medicare and Medicaid"), and moved out of state.

Now I hate Thursdays more than any other day of the week.

Ginger—Nadine told me the woman's real name again this morning, but it doesn't suit her half as well—asks Matt to push her chair right up next to the piano. *Closer, closer*, she trills. Tap, tap, tap, go those slippers, keeping perfect time with "Hello, My Baby."

Good-bye, my sanity.

Matt's eyes dart over to me; I let the drool I'd been saving for later dribble from my mouth. Ginger wipes my lips with the corner of her pink satin sleeve. The embroidery scratches my cheek, but I don't flinch.

Ted the Piano Man cracks his knuckles. He plays a brief flourish then takes us all down a notch. His next song will be "My Wild Irish Rose," and Ginger will eat it up.

CHECKOUT

Nadine is late today. I almost wonder why, but as she wheels me down the hall, past the rheumy gazes and limp finger waves of other Guests *en route* to the cafeteria (the Walnut Room), I spot the hearse (God's Special Chariot) parked outside the front doors, and I know.

I ponder the possible identity of the Passenger therein, and by the time Nadine sets the brakes on my chair, I have narrowed the list (based on the crowd of vultures sniffling by their rooms) to two: Big Mickey in 1C—the staff's nickname for him—and Judy Moody, across the hall in 1B.

I hope it wasn't her; she was the best show in the house. You can always tell when someone takes up cursing late in life: like someone learning a foreign language, they never quite get the hang of the rhythm.

Nadine settles in across from me and ties the bib around my neck. She works her spoon in my applesauce like an artist at a palette. I let her scoop, push, scrape, and wipe (Meal Assistance) until the tray is empty, never moving my eyes from her belt buckle to avoid accidental eye contact. I wonder if she knows the bottom button of her shirt is missing.

Later, as Nadine and I approach my room, I hear Ginger, whooping and laughing with her son and his family. Listening to the other residents' visitors here is like lying in a crowded maternity ward after you've just miscarried.

After Ginger's family (Our Special Guests) leave, the painfully yellow roses they have brought her will make me sneeze. I will let the snot drip down my nose until someone comes to wipe it away.

ROOM SERVICE

Ginger has insomnia. I know this because she told Nadine all about the "happy pills" that make her sleep. She takes them every night, and every night she snores and mumbles, cries and farts and hums loudly enough to wake the dead—except, sadly, for Judy Moody. Lucky Judy; the poster child for futile resistance has escaped at last.

Tonight, however, Ginger is quiet, but her mattress is squeaking, and that is what awakens me. I peek through the three or four eyelashes I have left and see Matt, bouncing up and down on top of Ginger.

His scrubs are down and her pink nightgown is up, and I know Ginger is too Ambien-scrambled to resist—or, likely, to remember. Oh, God.

I close my eyes, millimeter by millimeter, hoping my eyelids don't creak. I hold my breath and try to stop shaking. Nadine helped me use the bedpan before turning out the light, so I am utterly defenseless.

Matt grunts. After a bit of rustling, I feel his hot, beery breath over my face. Desperate, I form a bubble of sour, foamy saliva on my lips. He snorts and leaves.

SPA DAY

At breakfast, though Nadine straps my head up to prevent choking, when she asks me and Ginger how we are this beautiful morning, I choke on my oatmeal, spraying her. Nadine never gets angry when things like that happen, just gently wipes my face and her shirt. Her constant kindnesses to me almost make me feel I could tell her about what Matt is doing. But when she spins my chair around to face the TV and tells us Miss Carmen will be in soon to "make us pretty for Movie Night," instead of telling, I remember I can't count on anyone in here, and I belch instead.

Movie Night is a misnomer, since it takes place right before lunch, to give the sundowners among us a fighting shot at making it to THE END (of the movie). The staff wheels all the Guests into the Walnut Room Theatre—which they magically transform into a Graumanesque cinema palace by adding an oversized white screen and an Old Timey Popcorn Machine!—and lacerate us via a DVD from their rotating archive of Crap Designed to Make Old People Cry. It's quite the collection: *On Golden Pond, Cocoon, Driving Miss Daisy* are usually in heavy rotation. I last tasted popcorn several years ago, when a stray hull lodged under my dentures and caused an abscess. After that, they took my dentures away.

"Good morning, ladies. How are you?" Miss Carmen (Physical Therapist/Beautician) waddles behind her salon trolley into our suite.

"We're lovely, Carmen, how are you? What a beautiful morning, isn't it?" Ginger asks.

"Not as beautiful as you, gorgeous," Carmen says.

And so it begins—the relentless onslaught of silliness and tittering I will endure for the next hour while Carmen sets and teases Ginger's wig, trims and buffs Ginger's nails to a shine, and throws in some token range-of-motion exercises for Ginger's bursitic shoulder.

When she is finished with Ginger, Carmen turns on me, flourishing her gleaming scissors a couple of times over my scabby scalp for show.

"You know, I have so many wigs in storage at my son's house," Ginger says. "I could ask him to bring one."

I tongue the last slobber of oatmeal out the side of my mouth and pray, if not for Death, at least sudden-onset deafness, but as usual, both continue to ignore me.

Carmen wipes my face with a towel and continues our charade. "Aw, she's got a few curls left," she says. "No one sees her but us, anyway. There, all done, beautiful." She plants her customary sticky kiss on my cheek and drops her scissors as always. "I ought to put a bungee cord on these things." She grunts when she picks them up.

"Doesn't she have any family?" Ginger asks Carmen.

"She's got a son in California. He moved back out there a few years ago, as soon as he saw she was settled. Doesn't visit her but once a year now, if that," Carmen says, tucking her scissors back into her smock pocket.

"Oh, that's so sad," Ginger says.

"Disgraceful, is what it is," Carmen says. "But what can you do? Some families are just like that." She wheels her trolley to the door. "You ladies have a great day now," she says. The door hits her ample behind on the way out; I hear her muffled curse when the scissors clatter to the floor again.

Yes, Charles is "just like that" now.

At least he waited to show his true colors until after George died. I'm glad he's gone; seeing what our son has become would've killed him. I wish it could kill me.

DRIVE-IN

At ten o'clock, Renaldo (might well be his real name, though I'm not sure) parks the last body (Permanent Guest, head strapped up like mine) in front of the screen.

"Great, thanks, Renaldo," Matt says. "Hey, everyone, we have a big treat for you today, a *new* movie." Matt sweeps his girlishly long bangs back with his hand and holds up a case featuring the omnipresent image of Some Plucky Old Person(s) on the front. "Walter Matthau and Jack Lemmon, plus for you gents, Ann Margret. They don't come any hotter than her—except for my best girl over there."

"Come sit by me, Matt," Ginger calls out.

"It's a date," he says, flashing his pearly canines. He drags a chair over next to Ginger's wheelchair and drapes his arm across her shoulders. She sighs and snuggles her head against his arm. I want to scream at her. From somewhere deep inside me a feral, primitive urge starts my lips curling back from my empty gums. Nadine strokes me lightly on the shoulder.

"Shh, it's just a movie," she says. She's using exactly the type of soothing whisper I used to use with Charles, when he'd wake from his boyish nightmares.

Trying to cover for my loss of control, I force a loud gurgle from my throat. Matt turns his head and looks right at me.

I will have to be more careful.

BIRTHDAY SUIT

Carmen goes all out for my ninety-fifth birthday (Ten More Than Expected or Needed). At Ginger's urging, she buffs my nails, and bathes and lotions each accordioned inch of my body. To add insult to injury, she rakes the last of my curls together into a ridiculous pigtail on the top of my head.

"Look what I found for her," Carmen says to Ginger. "Isn't it sweet? They make these for little baby girls now. It's Velcro, so even if they don't have much hair, they can still have a pretty little bow."

She spins my chair around, and I glimpse in the bureau mirror a shriveled Kewpie doll, its head strapped to the back of its padded chair.

"Oh, that's just darling," Ginger says.

I've been pushing a slug of slimy mucus around the inside of my cheek with my tongue, and I wonder what would happen if I just spewed it at her, but Matt opens the door and again seems to look right at me. I gag on the gob as I choke it back down, and Ginger claps her hands.

"She likes it," she says.

Nadine wheels me into the Sunflower Room, where the staff has gathered all of the other Guests. Matt leads them in a stirring dirge of "Happy Birthday," and Ginger sings harmony.

When they did this to Judy Moody for her last birthday, she clawed the paper hat off her head and screamed, "Fuck off, you shit-fucking fuckers" to everyone, until they wheeled her, screaming, all the way down the hall to her room. I miss Judy Moody.

Nadine told Ginger Judy's son didn't even claim her ashes in person, just asked the director to ship them. I imagine Judy's vitriol-filled urn blowing the roof off the Fed Ex truck, and I almost crack a smile. At least I can count on my son to show up in person, as long as there's something to claim—car keys, bank books, family silver, wedding bands, ashes.

Being at the mercy of one's own child is a terrible thing.

Matt blows out my candles. Nadine nudges a little cake past my lips—scoop, push, scrape, and wipe—and then returns me to Ginger's and my room with Matt and Ginger hard on our heels. Nadine hums the birthday song to me as she pushes; she has a sweet voice. She pulls out my Velcro bow, along with a few more of my remaining hairs. I wince.

"Sorry," Nadine says, and gently rubs my scalp.

"She's a veg. Why apologize?" Matt asks.

Nadine reaches behind me and releases my head strap, supporting my chin as my head droops down. "Just because she doesn't talk or move so good doesn't mean she doesn't feel pain. And we don't know what she can hear, so try to be a little nicer, okay?"

I sense Matt studying me. I picture his shaggy head cocked to one side like a curious Golden Retriever, and I keep my eyes fastened on the calcified fingers curled in my lap.

"Okay, I'll be nicer," he says at last. His shoes turn away, and I can breathe again. He helps Nadine hoist Ginger into her bed beside the window; Ginger giggles and calls him her hero.

"Here, Matt," she says. "Would you please go in the top drawer of my bureau? There's a present in there from me."

"You know she doesn't know what's going on, right?" Matt asks.

"Maybe so, but she is my roomie. I asked my daughter-in-law to pick out something she would really like."

"How could you tell?" Matt says under his breath.

"Hush, Matt," Nadine says sharply over the sound of paper rustling. "What a beautiful scarf."

"Isn't it? I wasn't sure, because you can't see her eyes very often, but I think it will really bring out their color. Put it on." Ginger pushes the button to raise the head of her bed.

Nadine lifts my head and gently loops the scarf around my neck. She fiddles with the knot, trying to get it just right, then holds my head up, so everyone can see. I keep my eyes unfocused.

"There, I was right," Ginger says. "Look at those pretty brown eyes."

"Yep, those are pretty brown, all right," Matt says. I'd like to rip the scarf off my neck and choke him with it.

Nadine slips the scarf from my neck and folds it carefully. She helps me into my bed and plumps my pillows, then kisses my forehead. "Happy Birthday," she whispers before leaving.

Please, God, let this be the last.

EXPRESS CHECKOUT

Matt is in flagrante delicto when the Code Blue sounds. He leaps off Ginger, or at least he tries to, but the string of his scrub pants catches on her bed railing. There he is, half in and half out, hopping around like a hyperactive monkey tied to a grinder's organ. He gives the string a vicious yank and it rips loose just as our door swings open.

Renaldo does the tiniest of double takes when he sees Matt, standing beside Ginger's bed, retying his scrubs, but only says, "Yo, man, it's Big Mickey. All hands on deck. You all right?"

Matt brushes past him, running a hand through his hair. "Yeah, these shitty scrubs never stay tied." Their voices fade as they hurry down the hall.

Emboldened by a guaranteed staff-free twenty minutes, I lift my head from the pillow. My neck feels weak as a newborn's.

In the flashing Code Blue light, Ginger lies flat on her back, her knees splayed open against the bed railings and gleaming a sickly baby blue in the light from the alarm. The grotesque slackness of her jaw wallops me in the chest like a juddering fist, and goosebumps erupt all over my body.

Something on the table between our beds winks in the light. My muscles jerk and tremble as I lean closer on my elbow, watching Ginger and listening for the door. I recognize Miss Carmen's scissors.

I check the door and Ginger again. I begin rocking my body back and forth, thrusting my withered hand out as far as it will go, trying to build up enough momentum to reach the scissors. At last my fingers brush the cold metal; I grab the scissors and slip them into my pillowcase. Exhausted, I lie down again and wait, wait for someone, anyone, to come in and find Ginger Exposed, Ginger Violated, but no one comes. My tears dry on my cheeks, and I fall asleep thinking of Ginger, of Charles, and of Big Mickey. I wonder where they will find a big enough coffin.

PARTY LINE

Nadine comes in early the next morning. The moment she grasps the nature of the sticky residue on Ginger's inner thighs is violent and audible. She opens the door and yells for Matt.

"Hey, I was just leaving. I pulled a double and I'm beat," he says, sticking his head in the door.

"Look at this," Nadine says. She steps back from the bed so Matt can see Ginger, who is just coming around. "Did you see anything last night?"

"Whoa, what happened?" Matt asks. His gaze flits over to me and I go rigid. "No, man, we were busy last night. Mickey went, we needed everyone for that big elephant."

"Nice, Matt. Go get Dr. Lewis."

He bumps the foot of my bed hard on the way out. Inside my pillowcase, my fingertips seek out the handle of the scissors.

Guests and Staff start whispering almost immediately, and a parade of the concerned and the outraged, beginning with the Director, marches in and out of our room all day. I can't make out everything they say, but I pick up enough. One advantage of being a stone is they think you *can't* hear, so they don't realize you're always listening.

Nadine talks to Carmen, Carmen talks to Renaldo, Renaldo talks to Matt, Matt talks to Nadine, they all talk to Dr. Lewis, Dr. Lewis talks to Ginger's family, and everyone talks to the detective, who comes to visit directly after lunch. He looks like Columbo. Ginger, the fruity center of this entire mess, remains, incomprehensibly, her garrulously oblivious self, firing her undiluted charms point-blank at him as soon as he enters the room.

Everyone is talking, everyone except me; I know better. All the same, Matt's eyes, quick and sharp, grow warier by the hour.

GONE WITH THE WIND

Nadine squats down in front of my wheelchair. She leans way over so she can look up into my vacant eyes.

"You must've seen something, heard something. I wish you could tell us," she says, kneading my hand gently, her kind eyes imploring me to speak, speak. Waves of uncertainty wash over me. I think Nadine would believe me, but I'd be a pretty big damned fool to think she could protect me. The door opens, and my stomach turns over. The waves subside.

"Dr. Lewis is looking for you, Nadine," Matt says, coming to stand behind my chair. His breath heats the back of my neck, and I let my eyelids flutter close and noisily release my bowels, filling my diaper. Nadine jerks back at the sound.

"Jesus," Matt says.

"Yep, that's going to be a messy one," Nadine says. "I'll tell Dr. Lewis you said hi."

Before he can protest further, Nadine leaves. Matt makes a gagging noise, then leans down to begin cleaning me.

"Lucky for me you can't talk, I guess," he whispers in my ear. He lifts my gown and begins to whistle.

"AULD LANG SYNE"

Ted the Piano Man will be here tonight for a Special New Year's Eve (four to six p.m.) Gala. I gorge myself at lunch, flapping my open gums like a baby fulmar in the nest, taking every spoonful Nadine offers of creamed chipped beef, the finest culinary emetic, hoping not to attend due to illness, but no luck. Family members are invited, and some attend, but for most of the Guests, it's a night for remembering how alone we really are.

Ginger's family arrives early so her daughter-in-law can doll her up: a red, sequined top sporting a plunging neckline (Nadine calls it a Crumb Catcher); crimson lipstick; a fake poinsettia bloom pinned to her wig; and enough rhinestones to make a cowboy cry uncle. They bring me a red-sequined cap, too, which Nadine perches atop my strapped-up head and pronounces "festive."

When we enter the Walnut Room—which the staff magically transforms into a Winter Wonderland by adding a cardboard fireplace; strings of paper snowflakes sent to us by local schoolchildren (Community Service Project); and an Old Timey Popcorn Machine!—Ted the Piano Man is already in full swing, and, possibly, drunk. Nadine parks my chair close to the restroom. She hasn't trusted me as much since Columbo's last visit two months ago; when he couldn't ID the culprit, he eventually stopped coming around.

It's been quieter since then, though. Ginger must've stopped taking her Happy Pills, because she's started sleeping a lot less, and when she can't sleep at all, she reads trashy novels to herself in a stage whisper (I almost enjoy them). If she's awake when Matt sticks his head in, he just smiles and blows "his best girl" a good night kiss and leaves. I'm almost starting to feel safe again.

PILLOW TALK

The festivities finally end, the visitors leave, and we are put to bed early by a skeleton staff of broke volunteers and grumpy short-stick winners. I breathe a sigh of relief when everyone settles down and the floor is peaceful at last.

Shortly after lights-out, however, our door opens; the hall light silhouettes Matt briefly as he hurries past the foot of my bed to Ginger. The creamed chipped beef curdling in my gut suddenly decides to do its job as I envision him straddling her; I close my eyes and steel myself in preparation.

But something's different tonight in the sly rustling of the sheets, the flustered soughs of the mattress. I wait for the familiar catch-and-release of Matt's boozy breath when he finishes. Long moments pass, warped and silent. I tilt my head up a fraction of an inch, because I realize Matt is whispering.

"Hopefully you go faster than O'Brien did." He grunts in a way I haven't heard before. Ginger's bed frame rattles, making it harder for me to hear. I lift my head a titch more. "And Mrs. Rosenburg, shit." Another grunt. "Bitch nailed me in the nuts before she finally died—"

I can't stop my gasp, banshee-loud in this room. My mind races. *Mrs. Margaret O'Brien? Judy Moody? Does he mean he—*

Matt stops whispering and I freeze.

I am a stone, I am a stone, I am a—

"I knew you were in there."

I jump at the words so close to my ear, then the pillow slams down on my face. Matt's fingers dig into my nose through the pillow's thin spots, and his body presses me into the mattress. My wasted legs and twisted hands flutter up like broken birds. Bright stars erupt behind my eyes, a fiery galaxy of pain and infirmity, betrayal and abandonment, loneliness and degradation; my dying stars cool and harden, the vast black hole of me coming at last to swallow the world whole.

Hello, my baby, hello, my honey

Charles

I am a stone

I am a—

The pillow vanishes. Something strikes the bed hard and thuds to the floor, but I'm coughing and gasping and crying too hard to think what. My bright stars dim and flicker, blurring and diminishing until they coalesce into the form of Ginger, who is standing beside my bed, holding Carmen's scissors.

"Hello, there," she says, panting, a dark smear down the front of her pink nightgown.

I look around the room; there is a Matt-shaped lump on the floor between our beds. I can't see if it's still breathing.

"Are you okay?" she asks. She lowers herself onto my bed and whooshes out a Chanel No. 5-scented breath. The scissors dangling from her hand gleam stickily, drawing my eyes like a greedy fly to a honey pot. I lick my lips.

"They fell out when he grabbed your pillow. I snatched them," Ginger says. She drops the scissors on the table between our beds and wipes her hands on my blanket. Still confused, I glance down at her bare feet.

"Yeah, I'm stronger than I let on, just like you," she says. "Are you kidding? These legs?" She stretches them out before her and slaps them hard. "I could still dance all day," she says defensively. "What can I say? It gets me a little extra attention from my family. We do what we've got to do to survive, right?" The sudden hardness in her voice embraces me like an old friend.

We both look at the lump on the floor, which is stirring slightly. "You think a former Rockette doesn't know when someone's been after her? I'm old, but I'm no nun," she continues. She nudges Matt with her toes, and he groans. "Bastard. I suspected it was him, but I wasn't sure—too groggy. I started skipping pills, trying to catch him, since no one else would. I thought he might be in tonight for a little *auld lang syne.*" I am stunned. On the Mohs' Scale of Hardness, I realize, this woman would score an eleven.

"But Jesus, when he put that pillow over your face—well, I took care of it," she says, and that hardness turns to brittle pride. "All my life, I took care of myself. Good to know I still can." She winks, and I grab for her hands.

"Thank you," I say. My voice crackles like fresh exam-table paper.

A slow grin shimmies across her face. "I *knew* you were in there," she says. She leans closer, and her voice deepens to a fierce whisper. "Look, I don't blame you for checking out, for staying quiet. Being stuck in here is no easy thing."

Her eyes glitter like cracked-open geodes as she takes in our room: the matching hospital beds and wheelchairs and potty chairs; the gray walls festooned with monitors and tubing and cuffs; the bilious curtains hiding our view of the concrete parking lot and rusting dumpster outside. Her eyes come back to rest on Matthew, who is beginning to moan.

"Well." She reaches over me, pushes my call button, and returns to her own bed to wait for the help that will finally come. The rush of disappointment I feel at this surprises me; I lie back down and turn away from her to face the door.

"If you don't want me to tell anyone, I won't. I'll leave you out of it," Ginger says to my back. "But this is a tough place, especially alone. If you ever do feel like checking back in—" She leaves the invitation there.

I don't reply; instead, I use the seconds before the staff comes in and finds Matt the CNA (Cruise Director, Rapist) bleeding on our floor to weigh my options, such as they are in this hard, hard place. By the time the volunteer and the short-sticker, whose names I don't know, come running into the room, out of habit or out of fear, I am a stone once again.

Well, mostly.

GOLDEN ANNIVERSARY
KATIA D. ULYSSE

As I waited at the altar for you to walk down the aisle, the palms of my hands moistened, and my entire being trembled. I prayed that you had not had a change of heart, and my deepest wish would materialize before a hundred expectant witnesses. There was music. Soft. Fleeting. Piano? Maybe. I am not good at remembering details; you are the one who stores them like a baobab tree keeps water in its immense trunk.

Your brown skin shone under the Caribbean sun that never pretends to be forgiving. The bridesmaids smiled. The groomsmen hid their emotions behind stoic faces, but the tenderness in their eyes betrayed them. I was twenty-six. You were twenty-five. We were both full of life and ready to embark on our journey.

When at last I slipped the ring around your finger, I was transformed. Angels carried my breath on their wings during our first kiss as husband and wife, keeping me from drowning in bliss. There was applause when we danced our first of many dances. I whispered in your ears that on the day of our golden anniversary, we would dance like this—to the same melody.

You whispered, "This moment is all we have. Tomorrow is but a fantasy." I should have believed you.

When family members and friends tacitly boasted about their new cars, the house they lived in, and seaside residences with panoramic views of the distant horizon, I wanted you to have more. But you delighted in lacking ephemeral things, which tend to own people instead of the other way around. "We have each other," you said. "Our love is all the currency we really need."

You were not miserly, just sensible. You cautioned me never to float above my means. You predicted that the future—if such a time came—may be fraught with the unexpected. We would be prepared to face hard times bravely. As long as we stayed together, every battle would end in victory. There would be no regrets, only musings of extraordinary moments together.

I never imagined that on our golden anniversary rain would pour out of the sky, and catch us without shelter. For half a century, we weathered life's storms. We survived and even thrived. We were well-prepared, but we could not have known a nightmare like this would befall us.

The disease began slowly, almost imperceptibly. The doctors said it is not uncommon among people in their autumnal years. He said that at first you will not recall where you put the keys, and where you parked the car in the parking lot. But I was always the forgetful one. You were the one who would remind me to call my own parents on their birthdays long ago when they were still alive. You were the one who wrote textbooks and helped me organize my scattered thoughts. You were the one born an old soul—sensible and wise.

Now, you put the carton of milk under the kitchen sink. The eggs are on the bookshelf, and the cell phone is in the refrigerator. When we're supposed to go to bed, you open the front door—ready to wander into the night. You lose your way around the home we shared for fifty splendid years. And even though you're here, I fear I have lost you.

"Be gentle with her," the doctor says superfluously, as if I need to be reminded. Doesn't he know that I promised to hold and cherish you in sickness and in health? Doesn't he know I am a man of my word?

Today is our golden anniversary. The treasure trove of memories that always flowed from the wellspring inside of you has been ransacked, vandalized. When your eyes are not vacant, you stare at me as if I were a stranger. To be fair, I've changed. There are deep creases around my mouth and eyes, but I could not have changed so much that you would not recognize me.

Our life's savings of remembrances have been stolen. Your collection of ancient tales that were passed down to you like priceless heirlooms have dissolved into the thin and invisible air. You used to love talking about the history of your birth country. You could recount verbatim chapters from books about the only successful slave revolution known to man. We made pumpkin soup every New Year's Day to celebrate Haiti's independence in 1804. Now the holidays run into one another and hold no special meaning.

When people disparaged your birth country, you would hush them with the same detailed lectures you spent decades perfecting at the university. It pleased you to impart knowledge to thousands of wide-eyed students who adored you.

The history of beloved Haiti is no longer with you, is it? You've forgotten the names of the founding fathers and mothers. I watch as you search your mind for answers to questions you once formulated, but nothing comes. Our fifty years together have plummeted irretrievably into a murky pool at the bottom of a canyon, but I dare not ask you to reach that far into the unknown. It would not be safe. I would reach in, but my arms are useless unless you are in them.

The doctor says it's not unusual for someone with this condition to forget his or her own name now and again. Why should he expect you to remember your name, when I spent decades calling you *Sweetheart, Darling, My Love*—anything but the one on our marriage certificate?

Those hundred witnesses at our wedding fifty years ago are not here, but I am and always will be. There are no groomsmen today. No bridesmaids. I want to play our song, but I had trusted you to remind me of the melody.

I will wait for you at this altar in silence, praying that you will have a change of heart and emerge from the labyrinth where you reside now. I will wait until you return—if only for a brief moment—to dance with me to the rhythm of our hearts.

CONTRIBUTOR BIOGRAPHIES

Bari Diane Adelman is a writer with the soul of a social scientist, as reflected in her academic degrees. Her passion for observing and documenting the quirks of human behavior keeps her endlessly entertained. Whether she's writing about business, health, or family, she does it with true fondness and empathy for her subjects.

Malaika Adero is coauthor of *The Mother of Black Hollywood* by Jenifer Lewis and *Speak, So You Can Speak Again: The Life of Zora Neale Hurston* by Dr. Lucy Hurston and author of *Up South: Stories, Studies, and Letters of This Century's African-American Migrations*. She founded the book development firm and literary agency Adero's Literary Tribe, LLC. She lives in New York City.

Cathy Alter's articles and essays have appeared in *O, the Oprah Magazine*; *Martha Stewart Living*; the *Washington Post*; *Washingtonian*; the *Atlantic.com*; *Kveller*; and the *New York Times*. She is the author of *Virgin Territory: Stories from the Road to Womanhood*, the memoir *Up for Renewal: What Magazines Taught Me about Love, Sex, and Starting Over*, and *CRUSH: Writers Reflect on Love, Longing, and the Lasting Power of Their First Celebrity Crush*. A version of her story was published in *Washingtonian MOM*.

Jane Bandler spent thirty years traveling around the world as the spouse of a Foreign Service Officer, living in London, Ireland, Nigeria, Cameroon, Paris, Bonn, and Cyprus. During those various assignments and in Washington, DC, she pursued a twenty-five-year career as a Montessori Preschool Director. She retired to take care of her husband after his diagnosis of early-onset Alzheimer's disease and is the proud mother of three grown children and grandmother to three young grandsons.

Tina Jenkins Bell, a Chicagoan, writes short and long fiction, creative nonfiction, and plays. With two other writers, she recently created *"Looking for the Good Boy Yummy,"* a collaborative-hybrid short story that recounts the last days of Robert Sandifer, a young boy killed by his own gang (Black Lawrence Press, 2018).

Danielle C. Belton is editor in chief of the leading black website *The Root*. A St. Louis native, she has written in the past for the *Washington Post*, the *New York Times*, the *Daily Beast*, *Essence* magazine, *American Prospect*, and numerous others. A version of her story was published in *The Root*.

Cathie Borrie trained as a nurse in Vancouver and holds a Master of Public Health degree from Johns Hopkins University. She also graduated from the University of Saskatchewan with a degree in law, and she has studied creative writing at Simon Fraser University. She lives in North Vancouver.

Carol Bradley Bursack is a veteran family caregiver who spent more than two decades caring for a total of seven elders. She is a longtime newspaper columnist and the author *of Minding Our Elders: Caregivers Share Their Personal Stories*. She has also contributed to numerous other books covering caregiving and dementia.

Susan Kim Campbell is a writer of fiction and nonfiction. Her work is published in the *Alaska Quarterly Review*, *Meridian*, *SmokeLong Quarterly*, and the *Mississippi Review*.

Meridian commended her story as runner-up in their 2017 contest. Susan has been awarded artist residencies to the Millay Colony, Hedgebrook, the Anderson Center at Tower View, and others. She has won fellowships to the Writers @ Work Conference, the Tomales Bay Writers Conference, and the Norman Mailer Center. She holds a BA from Brown University. Visit susankimcampbell.com.

Meryl Comer is a cofounder of Us Against Alzheimer's, Women Against-Alzheimer's, and the Global Alliance on Women's Brain Health. From 2007 to 2019, Ms. Comer served as president and CEO of the Geoffrey Beene Foundation Alzheimer Initiative. She serves on the NIH National Advisory Council on Aging (NACA). She is a veteran broadcast journalist. One hundred percent of proceeds from her *New York Times* bestseller, *Slow Dancing with a Stranger: Lost and Found in the Age of Alzheimer's,* supports Alzheimer's research.

Edwidge Danticat is a Haitian-American novelist and short story writer. She is the acclaimed author of many books, including *The Dew Breaker*; *Breath, Eyes, Memory*; and *Brother, I'm Dying*. She has won many honors, including the American Book Award and the National Book Critics Circle Award.

Heather L. Davis is a mom, writer, and communications professional. She holds a BA in English from Hollins University and an MA in creative writing from Syracuse University, and has published poetry, fiction, and nonfiction in a variety of journals. Her book *The Lost Tribe of Us* won the Main Street Rag Poetry Book Award. She lives with her husband, the poet Jose Padua, and their two children in Washington, DC. She was deeply impacted by her time as an in-home caregiver for patients with Alzheimer's.

Miriam DeCosta-Willis is a former educator and author or editor of fourteen books, including *Blacks in Hispanic Literature, Erotique Noire/Black Erotica, The Memphis Diary of Ida B. Wells, Daughters of the Diaspora: Afra-Hispanic Writers, Notable Black Memphians,* and *Black Memphis Landmarks*. She cofounded the Memphis Black Writers' Workshop, was associate editor of *Sage: A Scholarly Journal of Black Women,* and editorial board member of the *Afro-Hispanic*

Review. In her forty-year career in education, she was the first black faculty member at Memphis State University and retired from the University of Maryland, Baltimore County.

Daisy Duarte is a patient and caregiver advocate for the LatinosAgainstAlzheimer's Network, bringing a valuable voice to advocacy, policy, and research discussions about the growing impact of Alzheimer's on the Latino community. Daisy is a caregiver for her mother, Sonia, who was diagnosed with early-onset Alzheimer's at age forty-eight. Daisy tested positive for the gene linked to early onset Alzheimer's disease in 2014 and is enrolled in the Dominantly Inherited Alzheimer's Network (DIAN) clinical trial at the Washington University School of Medicine in St. Louis. As one of the few Latinos enrolled in Alzheimer's clinical trial research, Daisy is committed to raising awareness of the importance of Alzheimer's research and funding. According to Daisy, "It's so important for Latinos and other minorities to engage in clinical trial research; we need to make sure that our communities have a voice in the research process. We have to take responsibility for our families and for ourselves."

Lauren Francis-Sharma is the author of *'Til the Well Runs Dry,* her first novel, awarded the Honor Fiction Prize by the Black Caucus of the American Library Association. She is the assistant director of Bread Loaf Writers' Conference and is currently working on her sophomore novel, to be published by Grove Atlantic in late 2019.

Lisa K. Friedman writes a regular humor column for the *Huffington Post.* Her other essays appear in the *New York Times* and in national and regional magazines. She has published two novels and eight nonfiction books. She lives in Washington, DC.

Lenore Gay is a licensed professional counselor with a master's in sociology and in rehabilitation counseling. She has worked in several agencies and psychiatric hospitals, and for ten years she maintained a private practice. Her poems and short stories have appeared in several journals. Her essay "Mistresses of Magic" was published in the anthology *In Praise of Our Teachers.*

Marita Golden is the award-winning author of seventeen works of fiction and nonfiction, which include *The Wide Circumference of Love* and *Migrations of the Heart.* As a cultural activist, she is cofounder and president emeritus of the Zora Neale Hurston/Richard Wright Foundation.

Evans D. Hopkins is the author of *Life after Life: A Story of Rage and Redemption.* He began writing as a member of the Black Panther Party Newspaper, under the editor-in chief, David DuBois. While serving twenty years in Virginia prisons for robbery and related offenses, Hopkins educated himself as a creative and political writer. He became one of the nation's most widely read incarcerated writers, with articles in the *Washington Post, The New Yorker,* and numerous other publications, and was paroled in 1997. He lives in Richmond, Virginia, with his wife and is working on a new book and other projects.

Julie Langsdorf is the recipient of four Individual Artist Awards in fiction from the Maryland State Arts Council. Her debut novel *White Elephant* was published by Ecco.

Cleyvis Natera was born in the Dominican Republic and immigrated to Harlem, New York, as a child. She has a bachelor's degree from Skidmore College and an MFA in fiction from New York University. She currently lives in Montclair, NJ, with her husband and two young children.

Elizabeth Nunez is the award-winning author of nine novels, including *Even in Paradise, Prospero's Daughter,* and *Bruised Hibiscus.* Her memoir *Not for Everyday Use,* excerpted here, won the 2015 Hurston/Wright Legacy Award.

Brendan O'Brien is a creative director at Small Army, one of Boston's top ad agencies. Before starting a career in advertising, he was an independent filmmaker, producing and directing documentary and narrative work. Brendan graduated from the University of North Carolina Wilmington in 2006 and lives in Boston with his wife, Laken, and their dog, Brewster.

Colleen O'Brien Everett graduated from Elon University in 2008 with a degree in communications and graduated from Notre Dame of Maryland in 2018 with a master's degree in Gifted Education. She is currently a teacher for Baltimore City Public Schools and lives in Baltimore with her husband, Matt, daughter, Adeline, and yellow lab, Crosby.

Greg O'Brien, author of *On Pluto: Inside the Mind of Alzheimer's*, is an award-winning journalist, a board member of UsAgainstAlzhiemer's, and an advisor to the Cure Alzheimer's Fund of Boston, and has served on the national Alzheimer's Association Early Onset Advisory Group in Chicago. He is the author of several books, has published eighteen books by other authors, and has contributed to national radio and television media such as NPR, PBS/NOVA, and others. Over the years, O'Brien has worked for major newspapers and publishing groups as a writer and editor and has contributed to *Huffington Post, Psychology Today, Boston Herald, Boston Herald American*, the *Washington Post, Time* magazine, *Chicago Tribune, Denver Post, Arizona Republic*, AP, UPI, *USA Today, Providence Journal, Boston Magazine, Reader's Digest*, and *Runner's World*, among other publications.

Joe A. Oppenheimer is an award-winning poet and fiction writer. His writing for adults focuses on injustice, loss, friendship, nature, aging, and the foibles of life. His work has been published in various literary reviews. "Charlemagne" first appeared in the fall 2016 issue of the *Corvus Review*. He was previously a professor of mathematical social science at the University of Maryland.

Julie Otsuka is the author of *When the Emperor Was Divine* and *The Buddha in the Attic*, which won the PEN/Faulkner Award and was a finalist for the National Book Award. She is the recipient of a Guggenheim Fellowship and an Award in Literature from the American Academy of Arts and Letters. Her work has appeared in *Granta*, *Harper's*, and *100 Years of the Best American Short Stories*. She lives in New York City.

Daniel C. Potts, MD, FAAN, is a neurologist, author, educator, and champion of those living with Alzheimer's disease and other dementias and their care partners. He was selected by the American Academy of Neurology as the 2008 Donald M. Palatucci Advocate of the Year. Inspired by his father's transformation in the throes of dementia from saw miller to watercolor artist through person-centered care and the expressive arts, Dr. Potts seeks to make these therapies more widely available through his foundation, Cognitive Dynamics.

Nihal Satyadev is the CEO and co-founder of the Youth Movement Against Alzheimer's (YMAA). In addition to his work with this nonprofit, Nihal has been an avid researcher of neurodegenerative diseases. He is currently working on assessing a correlation between Alzheimer's disease and periodontal disease.

David Shenk is the bestselling author of six books, including *The Genius in All of Us*, *The Forgetting*, *Data Smog*, and *The Immortal Game*. He is cohost of the public radio podcast *The Forgetting* and creator of the Living with Alzheimer's Film Project, and has contributed to *National Geographic*, the *New York Times*, the *Wall Street Journal*, *Nature Biotechnology*, *Harper's*, *The New Yorker*, the *Atlantic*, the *New Republic*, NPR, BBC, and PBS. Shenk lives in Brooklyn, NY, and Southfield, MA.

Julia Tagliere's work has appeared or is forthcoming in *The Writer*, the *Bookends Review*, *Potomac Review*, *Gargoyle Magazine*, *Washington Independent Review of Books*, *SmokeLongQuarterly*, and various anthologies. Julia resides in Maryland with her family, where she recently completed her MA in writing at Johns Hopkins University.

She serves as an editor with the *Baltimore Review* and is currently working on her next novel, *The Day the Music Didn't Die*.

Vicki Tapia, after teaching somewhere around ten thousand mother/baby pairs the art of breastfeeding, found her energies redirected to the other end of life after both her parents were diagnosed with dementia. A diary written to help her cope with caregiving morphed into *Somebody Stole My Iron: A Family Memoir of Dementia*, published by Praeclarus Press. Tapia's memoir was a finalist in the 2015 High Plains Book Awards. A sometimes blogger for the *Huffington Post*, she is currently at work on her second book and actively involved in the administration of AlzAuthors.com.

Sonsyrea Tate is the author of the memoirs *Little X: Growing Up in the Nation of Islam* and *Do Me Twice: My Life After Islam*. Sonsyrea has worked for the *Washington Post*, the *Chicago Tribune*, the *Virginian Pilot*, and several community newspapers. She currently works for the US Government Publishing Office.

Sallie Tisdale is the author of many essays and several books, most recently *Advice for Future Corpses*.

Katia D. Ulysse is a fiction writer, born in Haiti. Her short stories, essays, and Pushcart Prize–nominated poetry appear in numerous literary journals and anthologies, including: the *Caribbean Writer; Smartish Pace; Phoebe; Meridians: feminism, race, transnationalism; Mozayik,* the *Butterfly's Way,* and *Haiti Noir*. She has taught in Baltimore City's public school system for fourteen years and served as Goucher College's Spring 2017 Kratz Writer in Residence. She is the author of the critically acclaimed short story collection *Drifting.* Her latest novel, *Mouths Don't Speak*, continues to receive high praise from critics and readers.

Loretta Woodward Veney is the author of *Being My Mom's Mom* and *Refreshment for the Caregiver's Spirit*. Loretta is a motivational speaker and trainer who has delivered more than three hundred speeches and presentations on dementia and caregiving. Loretta and her mom have been featured in articles in the *Washington Post*, the *New York Times*, *AARP*, as well as a PBS special featuring Alzheimer's caregivers.

George Vradenburg is chairman of UsAgainstAlzheimer's, which he cofounded in October 2010. He was named by US Health and Human Services Secretary Kathleen Sebelius to serve on the Advisory Council on Research, Care, and Services established by the National Alzheimer's Project Act and has testified before Congress about the global Alzheimer's pandemic. He is a member of the World Dementia Council. He and UsAgainstAlzheimer's co-convene both the Leaders Engaged on Alzheimer's Disease (LEAD) Coalition and the Global CEO Initiative on Alzheimer's Disease. With his wife Trish (1946–2017), George has long been a dedicated member of Washington's civic and philanthropic community. George served as chairman of The Phillips Collection for thirteen years and is a member of the Council on Foreign Relations and the Economic Club of Washington. He has served in senior executive and legal positions at CBS, FOX and AOL/Time Warner. George and Trish published *Tikkun Magazine* for ten years.

Wren Wright, a former librarian retired from a global telecommunications company, holds a BA in communications-literary journalism from the University of Denver. Her writing has appeared in national and international literary magazines as well as local publications. Her ebook *The Grapes of Dementia: My Story of Love, Loss, Surrender, and Gratitude* chronicles her grieving process after her husband's diagnosis of early-onset dementia.

Ann Marshall Young retired from a career in the law in 2015 and since that time has focused her energies on community activism and service as well as writing. She has previously published articles on legal/ethical issues and her travels with women judges in China, and has now moved into the nonlegal arena, concentrating on personal/historical subjects.

ACKNOWLEDGMENTS

I want to thank my editor, Cal Barksdale, for his support and enthusiasm for this project. This is my second book with Skyhorse Publishing, and I have found the experience of working with the Skyhorse family one that continues to be deeply satisfying. This book is a project that was inspired by the commitment of the caregivers of those with Alzheimer's and dementia, those researching the disease and trying to find a cure, those living with it, those standing in friendship with those impacted by it. I wanted to provide a space where their stories—complex, surprising, troubling, inspiring—could be shared with dignity. The generous response of all the writers in this book has been gratifying. They have shared not only their stories but their networks, their communities, and their ideas for connecting these stories with the widest audience possible. Like nearly all the books I have written or edited, *UsAgainst Alzheimer's: Stories of Family, Love, and Faith* came to me as a surprise. Sometimes as a writer, you are "called." I no longer ask why. The dedicated, visionary team at UsAgainst Alzheimer's provided invaluable guidance along the journey from idea to book. I thank them for their service and hard work as Alzheimer's activists and for making this the fine book it turned out to be.

PERMISSIONS ACKNOWLEDGMENTS

I WON'T FORGET YOU

STRANGER THAN FICTION